I0129813

Foreword by Neil MacKinnon
BSc(Pharm), MSc(Pharm), PhD, FCSHP, FNAP

HEALTHY LOGIC

EVIDENCE-BASED HEALTHY AGING

GRAHAM C. MACKENZIE PH.C.

ULTIMATE PUBLISHING HOUSE

Copyright © 2021 by Ultimate Publishing House

Healthy Logic
Evidence-Based Healthy Aging
By: Graham C. Mackenzie PH.C.

All rights reserved as this book may not be reproduced in whole or in part, by any means, without written consent of the publisher.
For permission requests, write to the publisher, addressed
"Attention: Permissions Coordinator" at the address below:

THE ULTIMATE PUBLISHING HOUSE (UPH)
Canadian Office: 205 Glen Shields Avenue
Toronto, Ontario,
Canada L4K 2B0
Telephone: 647-883-1758

www.healthylogicbook.com

www.ultimatepublishinghouse.com
E-mail: info@ultimatepublishinghouse.com

Quantity discounts are available on bulk purchases of this book for reselling, educational purposes, subscription incentives, gifts, sponsorship, or fundraising. Unique books or book excerpts can also be fashioned to suit special needs such as private labeling with your logo on the cover and a message from or a message printed on the second page of the book.

For more information, please contact our Special Sales Department at Ultimate Publishing House. Orders for college textbook or course adoption use. Please contact Ultimate Publishing House Tel: 647-883-1758

Healthy Logic
Evidence-Based Healthy Aging
By: Graham C. Mackenzie PH.C.

ISBN: 978-1-7354831-4-6

HEALTHY LOGIC

EVIDENCE-BASED HEALTHY AGING

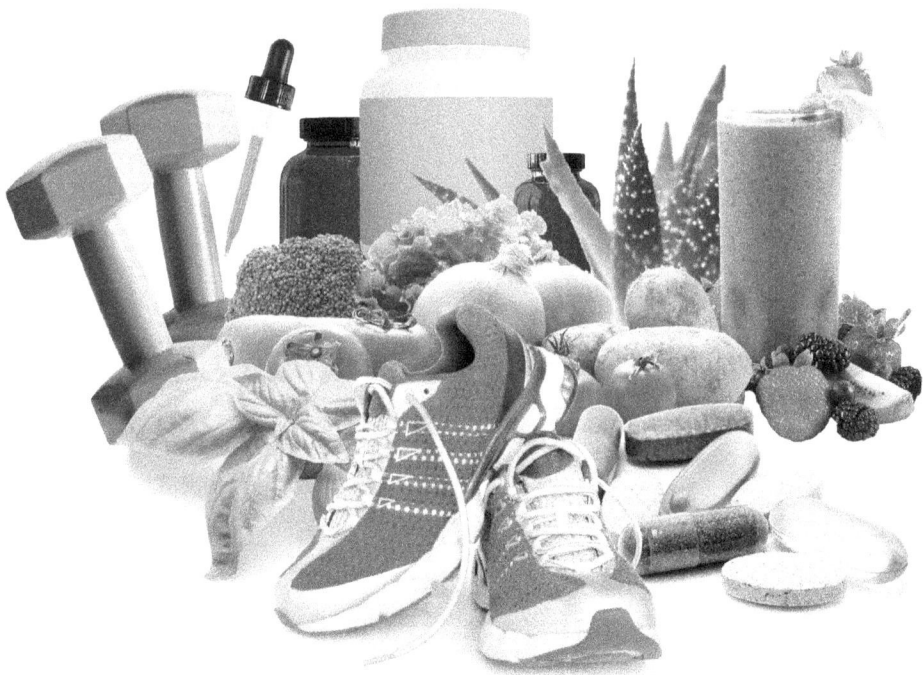

GRAHAM C. MACKENZIE PH.C.

To my wife, Bev.
When a good person contributes to the reasons for a longer life,
the reward is more time with them.

FOREWORD

Almost 30 years ago, Graham and I graduated together from the pharmacy program at Dalhousie University in Nova Scotia. In the three decades since then, Graham has provided health care to thousands of patients. A pharmacist and pharmacy owner in the beautiful Village of Baddeck in Cape Breton, he has become a national advocate for evidence-based medicine. He lives out his principles and beliefs in very real and practical ways, such as removing homeopathic products and sugary drinks from his pharmacy.

In *Healthy Logic*, the reader will gain valuable insights into evidence-based medicine, with a special focus on healthy aging. The book is packed full of practical advice and tips. As Graham mentions, the book is a 10-year labour of love. In it, he approaches healthy aging with a much wider lens then simply medications. With chapters on topics such as sleep, exercise, and healthy grocery shopping, a truly holistic approach to healthy living is presented. All readers will benefit from Graham's prescription for healthy aging.

—Neil MacKinnon, BSc(Pharm), MSc(Pharm), PhD, FCSHP, FNAP
 Provost, Augusta University, Georgia, USA and Professor, Medical College of Georgia

ACKNOWLEDGMENTS

A career of nearly thirty years in any profession doesn't happen independently. My mom and dad would subtly steer me toward career ideas at lunch and supper times (which were always together at the table). A career in astronomy didn't strike them as self-sustaining. When my dad died suddenly at 74, I took a keener interest in what makes us live to the age we do.

My first boss in pharmacy, Byron Sarson, was a keen influencer on my career. He owned a compounding store in Halifax while I attended Dalhousie University. Rarely a day goes by that I don't reflect on how he would handle a daily task that I find myself doing in my pharmacy. My compounding pathway was largely attributable to him. He would have his own words in this book had he still been alive today.

Dr. Frank Chandler was the dean of Dalhousie's College of Pharmacy while I was there. One of his tasks was to teach us about the world of supplements and the evidence for or against them. It was an interesting way of introducing conversations at the pharmacy to customers who were overwhelmed or confused over what they were hearing on the news or from friends. Considering the age of misinformation that was to come, it was a great introduction to relying on science.

To any educator, influencer, friend, family member, policymaker, or anyone who influenced my opinion on anything in this book, your input hasn't gone unnoticed. Hopefully, this attempt to show as much evidence as possible without overstretching conclusions will help you in some way.

TABLE OF CONTENTS

INTRODUCTION

As a pharmacist with nearly thirty years of practicing pharmacy, I am one of the key professionals on the healthcare team that you rely upon for your everyday care, such as your doctor, nurses, and possibly other healthcare practitioners such as a physiotherapist, a dietician, a doctor of osteopathy, or a psychotherapist. Other healthcare practitioners whose services you may use include a wide spectrum of providers in alternative healthcare such as a chiropractor, acupuncturist, hypnotherapist, homeopath, traditional therapist, Reiki master, yoga instructor, or naturopath.

As team members, pharmacists are the people you see when you are either sent to me by another healthcare team member or when you don't feel well and are looking for a solution.

I am also the person you seek when you are thinking preventatively about your health and wellness. Many people rely on their pharmacists for advice, direction, and solutions so they can feel good, heal from any ailments, and live their life more fully. As a pharmacist and member of your healthcare team, it is my job to keep you upright and healthy as long as possible. This may or may not include extending your lifespan.

While you may only see your pharmacist sporadically to fill a prescription from your doctor, we do much more. Pharmacists are trained to understand the whole body, including the mind, and which solutions are most likely to work for various concerns. In pharmacy school, we also learn about supplements, and for more than just deficiency issues.

As a customer, you give pharmacists like me your trust and reliance, for which I am grateful. We want to provide you with the best care you can get. You deserve it. The more we can educate you about your prescriptions and how to work preventatively against your ailments, the more we honour the trust you have placed in us.

The purpose of this book is to help you not only feel better, but also manage your own health care and lifestyle choices so you can live your best life, enjoy your family, and reap the resulting longevity that good health can provide. To earn your trust, I try to constantly stay informed about evidence-based care.

First and foremost, I am a pharmacist, educated in Canada and regulated by my provincial licensing body. Professionally and ethically, I am required to follow a given pathway of improving health outcomes using specific guidance. Getting to know your pharmacist allows both of you to become comfortable enough with each other to not only openly discuss your medical issues but for you to trust your pharmacist to follow best-evidence practices. Where the evidence is not as strong (as in much of the front-store environment), your pharmacist has the knowledge and is in a position to explain the various possible results of a treatment, so you will have a better understanding of whether it will work for you

After working in both large centres and a small village, I can confidently say that pharmacists are a trusted healthcare source in either setting. Positive patient-pharmacist relationships are essential everywhere, but in my village, since the next pharmacy is thirty minutes away, my reputation as a trusted healthcare provider and my relationship with my patients becomes even more unique and critical.

The internet and social media make it easier to have connections far and wide, and although the day-to-day recommendations may not be there, knowledgeable healthcare providers can still help others thousands of miles away. Whether advising patients locally or at a distance, a pharmacist's obligations are still the same: to improve the outcome in a health-related matter, not only with a specific recommendation, but also with a consistent philosophy of what you stand for and what you don't. As a provider of healthcare information to a larger population, pharmacists are obliged to convey a message that leaves a lasting impact of trusted evidence-based information. As a community member, your pharmacist has a responsibility to grow a stronger, healthier base of customers who think of that pharmacist first when it comes to accessibility of information.

Reflecting back on the ten years it took to write this book, I openly admit that for a while I was beginning to deviate from that path. Eliminating homeopathy and getting away from food sensitivity tests, unproven "nutraceutical" claims, and over-reaching recommendations on a host of medical conditions that didn't exist like adrenal fatigue and leaky gut were important. "Root cause" terminology and cherry-picked, poorly designed studies to back up over-the-counter recommendations became apparent. It soon became easier to understand one thing: medicine does not have all the answers, and making up therapies in an attempt to fill in these holes is a disservice to the patient. Ironically, the online national/international reach I just spoke of to drive home my own philosophy was the same method I used to steer away from suspect therapies.

So do all of my recommendations have a stack of studies behind them? Not really. Most over-the-counter meds don't have enough research behind them. Better studies are available with prescription meds, and lots of great references are there to back up therapeutic choices. But evidence is often on a continuum, where treating one out of four patients successfully is considered good odds. Studies often exclude patients for a variety of reasons. This leaves us to try and guess why a drug doesn't work for one patient but does for another. Best practices and good studies can back up choices, but there is never a guarantee in medicine.

Throughout this book, you will encounter my core philosophies. These include:

- Safety first, benefit second.
- Rely on evidence-based decision making.
- Lifestyle changes are often a good first approach.
- We cannot reverse aging, but we can help the odds of being upright longer.
- Sticking with science rather than gimmicks will serve you better in the long run.

The purpose of this book is to look at the medical and pharmaceutical treatments that our patients inquire about. We will also delve into the science behind the choices or the path that may have led our patients to seek out these treatments.

It's also critical to address the growing misinformation about various therapies, both under the self-care and physician-care categories. For example, the COVID-19 pandemic has taught us that human beings are not only willing to quickly accept unproven therapies, but they are also willing to promote these therapies to others. With the ease of the spread of misinformation on social media, we can see widespread use of an unproven product in the space of just a few days. Some recent examples connected to COVID have included hydroxychloroquine, ivermectin (an antiparasitic medication), and vaccine hesitancy.

Healthcare professionals accept that some people like to make their own decisions on healthcare, but at the same time we try our best to lay out evidence that has been proven through extensive studies. This is not a book about COVID or how best to treat it, but healthcare professionals are continually reminded of the barriers to correcting misinformation distribution, especially when it comes from seemingly reputable sources, such as healthcare professionals who are merely giving their opinion. An infectious disease expert may have a different, more informed recommendation than someone else in health care. It's important for all of us to pay attention to who is providing the information and where it is coming from.

In this book we will cover the full spectrum of human health. As a pharmacist, my first priority is to make sure my patients are not harming themselves with their choice or lack of choice of treatment. Ironically, the second priority is to figure out what works for them. You may wonder if these two priorities are reversed.

A WORD ABOUT OUR AGE-OLD FEARS OF AGING

How well we age is directly affected by the health conditions we experience. We clearly do not all age at the same rate. Differing variables like alcohol, drugs, smoking, exposure to second-hand smoke, stress, disease, diet, lack of sleep, obesity, environmental toxins, metal exposure, genetics, and the all-important exercise all affect our life expectancy. Each of these factors plays a part in affecting our DNA, the chains of information that make us what we are.

In order to age well, you need to become a partner on your own healthcare team. Don't get me wrong – none of us expect you to go to medical or pharmacy school and get a degree. But books like this provide you with the information you need in order to take charge of your life. I hope this book will empower you to become a stronger voice on your team and participate in the conversation about you and your health.

Please keep in mind that greater power comes with greater responsibility. Even though a doctor or pharmacist may not agree with you taking supplements or pursuing a particular route for your healthcare, you are responsible for informing them of what you are taking so they are aware of any potential interactions with their diagnosis, medicines prescribed, or other supplements that may be suggested. It's important to tell your medical professional about your daily habits, any meds or supplements you are taking, and your food choices, and how you are feeling.

WHAT THIS BOOK IS NOT

This is not an anti-modern Western medicine book. It is merely a guide to what evidence there is for the information we are inundated with daily. It is by no means meant to go against what your doctor prescribes. Perhaps your doctor is open to these ways of treating you, either in addition to or instead of his or her normal pathway. I see all points of the spectrum when I speak to physicians about what is considered acceptable "alternative therapy." Some feel "whatever works is fine with me," and others feel that medicine is medicine and anything alternative is not medicine.

If you are like most people, you are probably confused as to what you should or should not eat, or which supplements or over-the-counter or prescription medications might actually benefit you. Certainly, with the growth of the internet as a source of health information, I see many more people coming into my pharmacy looking for specific products than I did twenty-five years ago. Of course, there are some great sources of health information out there, but I often have to remind patients that they are looking at a tiny piece of the puzzle, while their physicians have access to a much larger picture. My goal is that by the end of this book, you will have a sense of what this larger picture looks like.

DISCLAIMER AND WHY TO READ THIS BOOK

Just like any other course of treatment, I recommend that you don't begin to take any over-the-counter (OTC) medication or supplements prior to consulting with a healthcare practitioner on your team. The recommendations in this book are not meant to diagnose, treat, or cure any disease. They are guidelines based on current cumulative science that is meant to contribute to a well-rounded, healthy lifestyle. They should be discussed with professionals on your healthcare team, which should help you boost your participation in your own healthcare efforts. It is my hope that after reading this book, you will be able to make a more educated guess yourself on whether the claim of a given treatment choice has any merit, and you will feel more confident and competent in evaluating information on the internet and talking with members of your healthcare team.

Reference: Hanna L-A, Hughes C. The influence of evidence-based medicine training on decision-making in relation to over-the-counter medicines: a qualitative study; *International Journal of Pharmacy Practice*. December 2012. Volume 20, Issue 6, 358-366.

HEALTHY LOGIC

CHAPTER 1

EVIDENCE-BASED MEDICINE

"We live in a society exquisitely dependent on science and technology, in which hardly anyone knows anything about science and technology."

– CARL SAGAN

As a patient, you rely on your healthcare team to support you, guide you, and determine your best course of action to attain, sustain, or, in some cases, regain optimal health.

You may or may not question a recommendation for care or supplementation from someone on your healthcare team. Sometimes you may seek out a veritable "assembly line" of professionals to help you, especially when you don't feel well. These professionals include your primary doctor, specialists he or she may recommend you see, nurses, pharmacists, dieticians, psychotherapists, and others who might be considered outside the realm of conventional medicine, including chiropractors, acupuncturists, physical therapists, massage therapists, and hypnotists.

Who you choose to rely on depends on whom you feel most comfortable with and in whose recommendations you feel most confident. Unfortunately, in this age of easily accessible information, it can be human nature to feel, after a few internet searches, that you are as knowledgeable as anyone on your healthcare team. It is also human nature to not only arrive at the conclusion you feel best suits you and your treatment, but to align yourself with the people who will help you pursue that treatment, even if it is not the best-informed decision or even completely wrong.

Generally, you spend the most time in the traditional "assembly line" with someone like me, the pharmacist. When you don't feel well, a doctor will prescribe something for you, or you will seek an over-the-counter medication such as a cough or cold medicine, a painkiller, or a vitamin supplement. Sometimes you may even choose a treatment based on something you have seen on television, read in a magazine, or found on the internet.

But how do you know whether these types of information are factual or "evidence-based"? Taking the internet's word for it doesn't always lead you to a pain-free path. In some cases, this approach can cause more harm than good. I want everyone to learn how to evaluate evidence behind a medical decision. In my practice, I attempt to make recommendations based consistently on evidence; that is what drove me to eliminate homeopathic products from my shelves.

HOMEOPATHIC PRODUCTS

I would never want to see someone walk out of a pharmacy with a homeopathic preparation for cancer treatment or prevention (or for any other reason, for that matter). I would rather recommend products that I believe, in my professional judgment, will work for the condition of the patient and hope they buy into that idea.

As a pharmacist, it is my job to tell someone if their medication choice is compatible with their other medications or medical conditions. I first thought these were a treatment option for those patients looking for an alternative, side-effect-free treatment.

As the years went on, I realized that homeopathic medicines were also results-free, evidence-free, and ingredient-free. I used to believe that if a patient included these products as part of their list of treatments, I would be the one to provide it to them. Back then, this option seemed better to me than having them go somewhere other than a pharmacy, where less professional individuals without a knowledge of the patient's medical history might attempt to upsell them or even recommend potentially harmful products.

The decision to withdraw homeopathic products from my pharmacy was not without opposition. Many of the people who visit my pharmacy or reside in the area were astounded by the withdrawal. The decision immediately sparked many discussions with patients at the pharmacy on what they could use instead of their homeopathic treatments. After making this decision, I was interviewed by a German magazine on this topic and found that the European continent has its fair share of homeo-believers. Some argued that they were getting relief from them. I argued it was placebo effect. Others wondered why I would remove something that some claimed gave results, even if it were placebo.

My response would be that it is unethical to give a placebo, charge money for it, and claim you helped a person with a medical problem when you really didn't. The danger in homeopathy is ignoring symptoms that may need real treatment.

Homeopathy belongs to a class of medicine often referred to as Complementary and Alternative Medicines or CAM. In the course of my career, I have had many debates with both patients and other healthcare providers about the validity of various types of treatment. Through years of practice, I have developed my own perspective of ethical decision-making in medicine – that perspective is rooted in what I call evidence-based medicine. Before I define this term, let's take a look at other types of treatments and approaches to medicine.

FUNCTIONAL MEDICINE

The idea behind functional medicine is that all the organ systems in the body should be treated as one unit. In this approach, a patient may not necessarily need a nephrologist, pulmonary specialist, or gastroenterologist. The claim of functional medicine is that all the organ systems are interconnected so strongly that the entire body should be addressed as one functioning unit, rather than a group of separate functioning units.

If you practice functional medicine and you are treating somebody who has anxiety or depression, you don't only focus on the brain or nervous system. You may also look at the gastrointestinal (GI) system or the patient's dietary habits and their nutrition. That is what functional medicine claims: each organ system has a function that contributes to the whole.

The unfortunate thing about functional medicine (and this is what gets it into trouble) is the lack of actual controlled trials that help determine the cause-and-effect claims that this type of medicine makes. In particular, functional medicine lacks trials that determine a cause and effect between treatments recommended by functional medicine practitioners and actual outcomes, such as increased lifespan or lowered heart attack rate.

Many people find the ideology and pathways of functional medicine to be attractive, but I have found that certain diagnoses that seem to stem from the field are problematic. Some examples might be leaky gut or adrenal fatigue. We often see a cluster of common symptoms and either apply a name to it or describe another "diagnosis" that needs to be fixed to cure it. When I hear diagnoses like these, I find they often have to do with marketing a specific product, as opposed to good, individualized treatment and medicine.

Critics of functional medicine often claim that it is merely a rebranding of the Complementary and Alternative Medicine that we mentioned earlier. Most traditional medicines that you may be familiar with fall into the wider CAM category. When we talk about traditional medicine, we are referring to all of the therapies and beliefs indigenous to different cultures, such as Chinese medicine and Reiki. Acupuncture and other forms of traditional medicine are not so much used by conventional medicine, or Western medicine, as I call it. Often traditional medicine also involves herbal medicine. More on the science we have on this later.

CONVENTIONAL MEDICINE

Conventional medicine is what you experience when you go to your family physician. We might also refer to it as "Western medicine." The organ systems are looked at individually and treated with each specific symptom in mind. There is a huge focus on bringing to market medical products that are backed by quality studies. Conventional Medicine also focuses on refining our current healthcare recommendations based on the same type of studies, as well as repeated case reports submitted by the professional community.

Having said this, conventional medicine has also been steered astray by the system known as "big pharma." The most notable example of this problem in recent decades was the pharmaceutical company Purdue and their push to bring their opioid pain reliever, Oxycontin, into the mainstream. The company downplayed their knowledge that addiction was a real problem with opioids. What resulted was a prescribing spree that is blamed for the opioid epidemic that we have today.

As an oversimplified explanation, conventional medicine says, "Here is your diagnosis, here are your symptoms or biomarkers. Here is the system affected and here is your medication." The medication referred to is the type I give out from my pharmacy every day. Treating by individual organ systems can result in overprescribing medications, particularly in the elderly, who cannot handle the medication load. As we will discuss in Chapter 6, most medications cause micronutrient deficiencies that result in side effects, and these side effects are treated with new medication. As a pharmacist, I spend a lot of time deprescribing, which is the collaborative effort of your healthcare team to remove medications from the list of drugs you take. Pharmacists often involve themselves in this practice. It can result in fewer prescriptions and a healthier patient.

EVIDENCE-BASED MEDICINE

Dr. David Sackett, commonly known as the father of evidence-based medicine, was born in Chicago in 1934 and became a Canadian citizen in 1974. He envisioned an evidence-based practice as not only using current best evidence but also individual clinical expertise. Duke University has outlined an evidence-based practice definition that involves making decisions for the patient, not based on evidence alone, but also using patient values and preferences as well as clinical expertise (or the clinician's experience, education and skills).

Although well-designed clinical trials are an important part of the decisions we make for patients, even positive trials have some subjects that didn't respond to the treatments they were testing.

What is our explanation for these patients? Inversely, could there be a correspondingly *small* percent of people that *only* respond to a given therapy when all others (the majority) do not respond fully?

Well-designed trials are inherently designed to kick these potentially important treatments to the curb and leave them in a "bunk bin" of treatments that are ridiculed and described as placebo, even when we know there are people for whom they work!

I pore through studies myself and read articles by trusted sources on reviews of virtually every treatment in the front of my store as well as in my pharmacy. This is known as following "evidence-based" treatment.

Another form of evidence-based evaluation on my part involves speaking to patients in my pharmacy. Thousands of such informa-tion-gathering sessions occur each and every year at the pharmacy counter and in the front store. Some critics feel this gives a jaded or misguided view of what works when contrasted with the results of well-designed scientific studies, but I vigorously disagree. Seeing real-time information from these patients and not using it would be a huge waste.

We know that clinical results shown to frontline healthcare professionals can take years to make it into official guidelines or mission statements. Such was the case with certain lice treatments that seemed to lose effectiveness over the years, almost like antibiotics. Pharmacists saw this happening long before the official word came out on it. It turned out to be true. As well, stool softeners rarely seemed to make much of an impact for most people taking them for constipation. Turns out, we were right. Still, they are widely used and recommended. I have spoken to many doctors, nurse practitioners, and pharmacists who have either a "go-to" list or an "avoid" list of treatments based on clinical experience with a treatment.

A key component here is the clinician's experience. It's hard to picture a physician who hasn't had a positive or negative experience with medication, which influences their decision in whether to prescribe it or not. Some prescribers may find that the stimulant laxative senna works in some of their patients and not others. Turns out that elderly patients with little to no mobility (like in a nursing home) rarely respond well to this type of laxative. Evidence is always being refined.

I recall an endocrinologist who once told me about a new insulin that they prescribed for a patient. One of the rare side effects associated with that insulin put that patient in the hospital. It took the clinician months to come around to prescribing this medication for patients going forward, even though the insulin was widely popular with other professionals. Clinical trials are a very important aspect of medicine but, in the end, whatever works for a particular patient is what should be prescribed for that patient.

Whoever you go to for treatment, whether they fall into the field of conventional medicine, functional medicine, or otherwise, I hope you ask questions to ensure that they are taking an evidence-based approach.

As patients, many of us believe that our treatment decisions are based on evidence that our healthcare professional has reviewed, read, or been taught in school. We often don't review the studies ourselves.

As we will see, evidence presents itself to us in many ways; the key is to realize how reliable or unreliable that evidence is and how to avoid total reliance on anecdotal evidence or personal beliefs.

BAD EVIDENCE

The doctor you see doesn't always have time to review and read all the studies about a particular medication when the representative from the pharmaceutical company comes in with all their charts, research, and studies. The busy doctor often has to process it quickly and says, "Okay. I'm willing to prescribe this to my patients." There is a huge reliance on the government regulation arm, in my case Health Canada, to police what the drug company does.

Unfortunately, there is little burden of proof put on the company if it is an over-the-counter (OTC) product. There is more of an effort put into making sure the product is not directly harmful or contaminated. Sometimes the physician or nurse practitioner who recommends a product to you will attend conferences that bring together all available consensus and information on ways to treat a given medical issue, and that may include drug recommendations.

For products we regularly provide over the counter, from medicines for coughs and colds to products for constipation and hemorrhoids, we pharmacists go by what we were taught in school and what we learned in continuing education or clinical experience. That is an important third component.

If "evidence-based" means taking all of the evidence available and applying it to practice, then this means avoiding the urge to rely strictly on the last study done, with ground-breaking controversial results that make it to the media.

Sadly, it is commonplace for a study to be misrepresented in the media, spreading misinformation on treatment or lifestyle interventions. It is important to realize that the conclusion of a scientific study can only confirm or deny specifically what it has tested. Speculation and extrapolation are great drivers of future research, but they do not belong in the conclusion of a research paper or in the headline of the newspaper.

It is also important to resist the urge to nullify previous studies just because a new study seems to contradict older ones. A full understanding of the truth comes from adding the new study to all of the previous ones, like a puzzle. Extra attention is brought to a study that duplicates findings of a previous one, as it strengthens a previous finding.

When we sift out the well-designed studies from the others and recognize the power of each study and what it is are capable of telling us, we are left with a vast and valuable bank of information to guide treatments.

We have several modalities of information-gathering available to us. In medicine, we are always striving to reach the 100 percent truth out there somewhere in infinity. We are always striving for the full puzzle to be completed.

Let's examine these modalities:

TYPES OF EVIDENCE – DNA

Our DNA is for the most part the same for everyone, except for a small number of differences. Some of these differences are obvious and visible, like our hair colour or our height. There may be other changes inside of us that determine our response to medications. The main job of our DNA is to create messages that are used to make proteins in our body that carry out most of the work the body does to survive, reproduce, and develop.

DNA is also responsible for determining how each of us respond to the world. We don't all respond equally to the same medication. This is something we see in medicine all the time. There are many possible reasons for this. In some cases, there may be subtle but important variances in our DNA that require a different daily amount of a single nutrient or medication. There are already tests available to indicate if you are an outlier in the way you respond to various types of medications. Although not widely used yet, such tests have the potential to head off a trial-and-error approach to medications such as antidepressants. Tests are also available with genetic counselling that can give you information on your chances for various diseases like Huntington's disease and even cancer. It's important to note that while your diet, nutrition, and exercise are all important in your DNA's health and your longevity, disease and life expectancy are complex issues that often rely on multiple factors.

DNA is mainly found in the nuclei of our cells and, to a lesser extent, in our cells' mitochondria, where our chemical energy is produced. This remarkable chain of biochemical information is tightly and efficiently coiled in a double helix formation of chromosomes, which each contain a specific number of genes. They carry so much information that a single cell's DNA would extend about two metres. When a cell in your body divides to create a new cell, the double helix effectively "unzips," and each one duplicates to provide a brand-new pair of helix for the new cell and one for the old cell. In this process, there are safeguards against errors in duplication, but they still can occur.

Differences in nutrient requirement, medication response, and disease susceptibility are often the result of small "typos" called SNPs or snips, which occur when the DNA duplicates in preparation for cell division. SNPs (single nucleotide polymorphisms) are the most common form of genetic variation among humans. Most of the time, these typos have little consequence, but they can lead to one person having a different response to a medication compared to another person, or a different susceptibility to diseases like heart disease, cancer, or diabetes. There are hundreds of millions of SNPs found in humans in differing populations and help explain why certain diseases are more prevalent in certain populations. Ironically, we can now use gene sequencing to treat cancer that was caused by the DNA in the first place. Sequencing is when we determine the order of the four basic building blocks called bases that make up a DNA molecule.

Some patients complain that they just can't seem to tolerate any anti-inflammatory pain relievers or any antidepressants. It turns out that these patients may actually be correct. Just because we cannot explain something doesn't mean it's all in their head. Genetic testing could be important for many individuals to save time and money and prevent side effects. SNPs are passed down to your children and their children and help explain why certain diseases or individual responses to drugs run in families.

At a pain and addiction conference where I once presented to a group of physicians, I introduced the concept of hereditary SNPs and how they relate to opioid misuse. I don't recommend testing everyone for their metabolism of opioids before they start on them, but for those who don't respond at normal doses, it helps to give a clearer picture. There are patients who are taking codeine for pain that metabolize it so slowly into its active form that they would need ten times the regular dose to achieve an effect.

Codeine is a pro-drug. This means it is metabolized by the body after the drug is absorbed to the active form – at which point the patient may be overloaded with active drug if too much was taken because the patient thought it wasn't working. Conversely, there are those who metabolize it so quickly into the active form that they are sensitive to even the lower end of regular dosing. Genetics is a significant determinant of which way you metabolize.

Our genetics even determine the activity of our receptors in the cell membranes that greet the opioid and result in the pain-relieving response. Medication will always be more than just swallowing a pill, with all of us hoping to get the same response as everyone else.

Now that we understand how genetics can affect how we metabolize nutrients and pharmaceuticals, let's discuss how it influences the instance of disease.

GENETICS AND DISEASE

You are not always destined to have a disease because of your genetics. You have some influence on how this part of your DNA shows itself to the outside world. Everything you eat, breathe, and absorb into your body is used as a signal to your cells.

Instead of our bodies being controlled randomly by a mindless DNA computer from the inside out, our bodies are fine-tuned by the contents of the fluid-filled space surrounding all of our cells called the extracellular matrix. This matrix is a reflection of our immune system, our state of inflammation, our stress levels, our cellular damage, and our bad and good habits.

The molecules and nutrients in the extracellular matrix meet with each other and with the membranes of the cells in your body and cause changes inside your cells. Molecules either directly passing through the membrane or causing a chain reaction without actually passing through all have an effect inside the cell.

Once this reaction occurs, and the signal has "translated" itself into the intracellular fluid (inside) of the cell, various steps can occur inside and outside of the nucleus of the cell, resulting in a different response from that bag of chips you just ate or the green smoothie you just drank.

An analogy would be something like this: If I was mowing the lawn and wanted a drink of water, I have two options. I could go into the house (cell) myself or I could ask my son (messenger on the cell membrane) to tell my wife that I need the water. Getting the water is a desired effect. If I didn't speak the same language as the messenger, or the door to the house was locked and I couldn't get in, this would represent a DNA change that challenges the action getting done correctly.

For the most part, you are everything you are because your DNA says so. Your DNA is like a semi-rigid piece of clay that is continually molded or expressed into something different, based on what it is told to do. It responds to the environment we present to it. We are all human, but our DNA is not all the same. For example, the colour of our eyes, hair, and skin vary. We are all different shapes and sizes and have different personalities. Some of us have diabetes, heart disease, chronic pain, different basal metabolic rates, high blood pressure, or thyroid problems. Some have arthritis, cancer, lupus, metabolism issues, depression, anxiety, ADHD, allergies, or gall bladder problems. In short, we have disease and discomfort. Though it is certainly not the only factor, genetics can predispose us to any of the diseases I have listed above.

When you take a step back and look at the bigger picture of all influencers affecting your DNA, we witness a universe of complexity.

With genetic research, we have an entire universe open to our eyes that we have only begun to see clearly within the last one hundred years. We are now getting a clearer picture of which genes are responsible for which processes. As the cost of genetic mapping steadily decreases, DNA will become more important as a form of medical evidence in the coming decades.

TYPES OF EVIDENCE – STUDIES

Academic studies are another form of evidence available to healthcare providers and practitioners. Healthcare professionals gain new information through journals and education courses and from pharmaceutical representatives who bring them the latest and greatest studies along with their products, in the hopes that the physicians will prescribe them. You as a patient often don't hear about these studies and, more often than not, you don't ask about them. You rely on your healthcare provider to know about them and provide you with a recommendation for your health condition.

There are a variety of studies out there. Some are more reliable than others. Some provide less scientific research but still add value for healthcare providers determining how to best prevent and treat diseases. There are case reports, cohort studies, meta-analyses, cross-sectional studies, epidemiological studies, and double-blind placebos. There are also natural studies that are done spontaneously in certain locations or environments by people who want to test a theory.

Randomized Controlled Trials
Randomized controlled trials are the standard by which we try to find out the truth. The key that unlocks the information from these trials is called statistical analysis. It helps determine if what we are seeing from our observations is by chance or is actual non-random results.

Randomizing means all subjects are randomly assigned to either a placebo group or an active group. We may have a screening process for inclusion of subjects into the study so we have a cleaner picture of our results, so subjects are not often randomly grabbed off the street. They are randomized after that point, however. For example, if the study has a comparison group that uses a placebo, the study subjects are randomly assigned to either that group or the drug group.

Statistical analysis has the power to take your information from a study (the data) and mathematically determine if the results from the control group (also known as placebo or "sugar pill") are sufficiently different enough from the active (drug) group based on the number of patients tested with the actual drug (or N number) to be an actual benefit of the drug and not from random chance.

Let's look at an example to understand some of the basic foundations of statistics. If I flipped a coin ten times, I may get tails seven times and heads three times. Now, using logic, assuming that the coin never lands on its edge, we know that the chances of it landing on heads or tails is 50%. Why did it show tails 70% of the time? The answer is because as we toss the coin more times, the number of heads and tails will gradually even out to close to 50% each. This demonstrates the increased power of study by increasing N, or the number of tests done within that experiment.

Anecdotal Studies

A conclusion that is drawn from an N of one study, or a one-patient study, or from a very small sample size, like a family of 5 people (N of 5) is usually referred to as anecdotal. Anecdotal studies are usually considered to be unscientific. If Aunt Mary took a certain supplement and it worked, does that mean that actually it worked for her, or was it just by chance that she improved? Science says you cannot say with certainty. Pharmacists, however, are used to seeing these N of 1 situations multiple times every day. While anecdotal evidence about what has helped to relieve the symptoms of a single individual like Aunt Mary can lead many consumers astray, pharmacists are in a difference position. All of our patients' N of 1 anecdotes are gathered into a mental database that we call our "clinical experience."

Double-blind Placebo-Controlled Crossover Trials
Double-blind placebo-controlled crossover trials are the gold standard in scientific research. In these studies, the "double-blinded" trials mean neither the researcher measuring the results nor the subject receiving the drug or placebo knows what they are getting. This eliminates subjective opinion and provides as much objectivity as possible to the results.

The placebo, being the "sugar pill" or blank medication given, is important because "placebo effect," or a change in observation when a pretend pill is given, is a real physiological phenomenon. It can even be seen with infants and pets and even plants.

The perceived benefit of the caregiver or the assumption of being given a medication is a strong driver of the placebo effect. This needs to be compared to the change in effect when the real medication is given, and the difference must be applied to statistical analysis.

Crossover trials will apply a placebo and test drug for a while and then switch groups to see if there is a change in the effect. They may even switch placebo and control groups back again to verify the change. As an added benefit, some studies use more than one location or are multicentre in design. This can have the added benefit of minimizing bias or improper technique in one lab as opposed to all of the other labs.

If the centres are widely separated geographically, we can also see differing results based on inherited differences within a certain area that may not be in another, resulting in differing responses to the medication.

So, depending on the funding a particular study has, it may have the ability to apply these strategies to strengthen the power of the study to make a claim in its conclusion. Ironically, the source of the funding can also be a weakness in a study, especially if it is supplied by a party with a vested interest in the outcome.

Case Reports

Case reports are among the weakest statistically, because there is no control or placebo group to compare them to. Having said that, I have spoken to many physicians who have had a good or bad experience with a medication one time that can significantly impact whether they prescribe that medication again. There are also case control studies where someone is compared to others who don't have the same medical condition. In this type of study, we compare which factors were different with that person compared to the others and why that led to the development of the medical condition in that person. These studies often lack a randomized procedure and cannot come to a firm conclusion as to what caused the disease in the first place, but they are interesting in that they can direct future research toward finding the origin of a disease.

Cohort Studies

Cohort studies follow a group that has been exposed to a variable and compare them to another group without that exposure. These are strictly observational and again do not hold the reliability of the randomized controlled studies. The biggest source of error in cohort studies is that there could be many differences between the two groups that we don't know about, which affect the outcome. A retrospective cohort is similar, except data on the subjects in the study is researched from their history. When you see the word "prospective," it means that the data was collected over time from the beginning of the study, starting before the outcome of interest occurs.

Cross-Sectional Studies

Cross-sectional studies are like a CAT scan of a group that shows a trait in that group compared to another group. For example, the vitamin D levels in people who live near the equator as compared to those who live at a higher latitude, and why the incidence of multiple sclerosis (MS) is lower at the equator. Another example is why "Westernized" countries around the globe have a higher incidence of certain types of cancer relative to other countries and the correlation between these countries' higher cancer incidence and certain dietary similarities such as low omega-3 intake in the food.

Epidemiological Studies

Epidemiological studies look at the distribution of a disease and any changes over time in disease frequency, as well as what might be causing those findings. These studies can be observational (cohort, case control, cross-sectional ecological studies) or experimental in nature. Cause-and-effect relationships are implied but need to be proven by more rigorous methods. It is important to take note here that the entire "stop smoking" campaign was initially based and is still largely backed by this type of study. As much as the epidemiological study has been criticized for not having certain conclusive powers, it certainly proved itself in that instance and saved many countless lives and extended lifespans immensely.

Meta-Analysis

A meta-analysis is a common type of study design where a search is done of other studies already completed on a similar topic. The data is extracted from these studies and gathered into one large group of data and reapplied to statistical analysis.

Meta-analysis is an interesting way of applying old data to a new study, but any shortcomings in the studies it draws the data from are carried forward into its results and conclusions. These types of studies are valuable in that you can weed out bad studies and focus on specific characteristics and study styles.

Similarly, a systematic review does research to find well-designed studies that help to answer a specific question based on the cumulative results of these other studies. The difference between the two types of studies is that a meta-analysis summarizes results of studies, whereas a systematic review aims to answer a specific question by looking at previous data. The Cochrane Database has systematic reviews for many topics of health concern for both health professionals and the public to read. You can imagine the power in these types of analyses, especially when a meta-analysis is done on other meta-analyses!

As you can see, there are many ways of following the scientific method to answer our questions, and there are actually more that are not mentioned here. The key is to realize the limitations and strengths of each method, and how they are able to contribute to medical recommendations that are science-based. It is important to remember that one study doesn't educate you on a topic, but it can be an important puzzle piece. The goal of science is to make clear the difference between a decision based on belief and one based on scientific proof. In the time we've been fighting COVID-19, the evidence has changed quickly, resulting in rapidly changing recommendations from good and bad sources. When it comes to your health, it's best to make decisions based on scientific proof rather than on social media opinions.

British physician and science writer Ben Goldacre describes placebo-controlled trials as a less effective way to further our knowledge of medicine. He suggests that comparing the study's medicine to the currently most effective medicine is a better way of furthering our knowledge, rather than comparing it to a placebo, which should be doing nothing. He is also a huge proponent of completely open access to all data in all trials, rather than the sugar-coated ones that make their way to Health Canada, the FDA, or the sales rep presenting data in the doctor's office.

The main takeaway message is that just because a study shows up on your newsfeed does not necessarily mean that it is gospel. Sometimes it is, but the general public is often in the dark about the accuracy of the claims and conclusions of any scientific study.

EVIDENCE-BASED MEDICINE IN TODAY'S SOCIETY

To stay well, you should consider where you are getting your information, evaluate its level of truthfulness, and make decisions about your mediations, your diet, and your daily habits so you will live as healthily and as long as possible.

Let me help you better understand what choices you have, what dialogues you could be having with your healthcare practitioners, and how to best attain and maintain optimal health.

CHAPTER 2

NUTRITION AND GENETICALLY MODIFIED ORGANISMS

"Fairness forces you – even when you are writing a piece highly critical of, say, genetically modified food, as I have done – to make sure you represent the other side as extensively and as accurately as you possibly can."

– MICHAEL POLLAN

A major factor associated with your overall disease state is your nutrition. Nutrition is initiated into the body by tasting the food, but after that what happens? Do your cells or organs taste the food and respond to it? Of course not. Extracellular matrix theory states that nutrition or lack thereof is a signal to the cells of your body. Nutrition creates the milieu that bathes your cells. This is the environment around and between the cells that make up the human body. It communicates the nutrients in your meal to the DNA in the nucleus of your cells. This communication connects the food you eat to a process in your cells at the molecular level to run the thousands of pathways that not only keep you alive but have a role in the possible development of cancer, infection, diabetes, mitochondrial dysfunction, or an autoimmune condition.

Why does one identical twin die of cancer at age fifty and the other from a heart attack at seventy-five? Well, maybe it's more than a predisposed DNA sequence. We are exposed to multiple insults on a daily basis as well as multiple props to enhance (note how I avoided the word "boost") our defense mechanisms. "Insults" is a general term we use to describe inputs that are likely to have a detrimental effect on human health; for example, certain chemicals, heavy metals, radiation, physical injuries, xenoestrogens, and viruses and bacteria. In today's world, all of these are pretty difficult to avoid. The opposite side of the health equation is stacked by your genetics (DNA), your nutrition, and positive lifestyle choices that give your body's cells the ability to assemble defense mechanisms needed to fight off insults. Socioeconomic status can also affect diet and exercise; therefore, disease state and overall longevity, independent of genetics.

It may be that, in the last few generations, we have allowed this health equation to become unbalanced. Eating whole food a few generations ago has slowly been replaced by a different way of eating, with more processed and ultra-processed food with less nutrient value. Weigh this loss of nutrients against an increase of insults that has occurred since the dawn of the industrial revolution and the subsequent rise of industrial agriculture. Insults are additive. For example, if I asked you to hold out your hands to catch marbles that I was dropping, initially you would have no problem catching all of them. As your hands become full, however, you might drop one. This represents the final insult over a lifetime of additive insults that, individually, seemed to not cause any problem. The better your DNA, nutrition, and lifestyle choices, the bigger your hands.

What about the seventy-year-old lady who smoked since she was fifteen? Perhaps she balanced the other side of the equation by eating a healthy diet most of her life and was blessed with genes that did a good job of assembling the body's natural defense mechanisms. Or maybe her genes rendered the dangers of smoking as harmless.

Organic food is often downplayed by modern medicine because the amount of conventional food with pesticide you need to consume to have an issue is so large that statistically it is a non-issue. Although I have an organic and non-Genetically Modified Organisms (GMO) section in my pharmacy, I do not feel it is particularly unhealthy to eat regular food that is not from this section. I simply offer it because the demand is there, and it is safe.

This is my feeling with all of the daily "insults" I listed at the start of this chapter: Why wouldn't you want to keep the number of marbles as low as possible? When I stopped selling sugary beverages in my pharmacy, I was often asked if I ever drink pop or juice. Did I think it would kill someone to drink one glass here or there? To me, sugary beverages and the nonorganic food are all lumped in the same bag of marbles with automobile exhaust, heavy metal exposure, cigarette smoke, fertilizers, pesticides, herbicides, dry cleaning fluid, and so on. The more you restrict the bad stuff, the more you preserve your health – incrementally!

SOCIOECONOMICS

This is as good a place as any to pause briefly and talk about socioeconomics. One overarching fact in keeping our health and preventing long-term disease is that these issues have both everything and nothing to do with medications, supplements, exercise, stress, smoking, or diet. The greatest common denominator in health and disease is often low income. The poorest people in my community are not buying from my organic food section. It is difficult for someone who lacks the economic wherewithal to have proper nutrition, safe housing, and social connections to show up on the statistics list of healthy citizens. While it is important for a government to promote healthy eating and exercise, perhaps their efforts to produce a healthy population should focus more on reducing poverty and increasing education.

No matter what your socioeconomic status, my wish for you is that you think carefully about the inputs that enter your extracellular matrix. You do not have to be rich to eat healthy foods. Each of us has very little idea of the exact strength or predisposition of our DNA in regard to disease. But we can all increase our chances of living a long, healthy life by eating right, exercising, and avoiding inflammation triggers and stress. Regardless of your DNA and genetics, living this way will improve your life expectancy.

NUTRITION AT THE PHARMACY

In my consultations with patients, I invariably make certain broad recommendations about diet. As a pharmacist, I recognize there are dieticians who are the experts on this topic and I encourage people to consult with one. You will not find overly specific recommendations here or at my pharmacy for that reason. My recommendations lean toward the new Canada Health Guide in broad strokes. For example, just entering your local grocery store, the first section you probably come across is produce. Here we find the least processed food in the store. Food as nature intended, with the exception of all of those genetically modified organisms, fertilizers, pesticides, and herbicides.

Patients in my rural area often expressed the desire to try to eat organic whenever possible. As a healthcare professional, I was encouraged, as seeing a patient motivated to eat right is half the battle. Following this, when celiac patients expressed concern on the availability of suitable food, out went twenty-four feet of magazine aisle and in came organic and gluten-free food. I am not one to think the entire world absolutely needs to be gluten-free, but some people express the desire to eat this way. Being partly in control of this choice by guiding healthy food choices turned out to be more of a challenge for me than I might have anticipated early in my career.

THE SUGARY BEVERAGE STORY

"Avoid sugary beverages, including pop, juice, and vitamin water." This was another common recommendation. I would watch customers leave the pharmacy, walking past these pop coolers. The irony was not lost on me. One day, I decided to remove the coolers and their contents, a move that seemed innocuous enough. The decision resulted in a few days of local and national news coverage and a flurry of interviews and comments on social media, mostly all favourable and supportive. There were a few "nanny state" remarks. A discussion or two arose about the possibility of an extra tax on sugary beverages. Of course, some were against this as well. I don't really see a sugary beverage tax as the government being overprotective or interfering, any more than a toll on a bridge or highway to cover expenses is "nanny state." It simply helps to pay for the extra expenses incurred from obesity-related costs in the medical world. Was the fact that I wasn't selling them anymore going to prevent people from buying pop and juice? Not really. They could just go up the street and buy it. As we will see, it turns out they didn't.

The decision to eliminate pop coolers from the pharmacy had another positive effect. It inspired a research study led by Leia Minaker and her team at the University of Waterloo. (Minaker LM, et al. An Evaluation of the Impact of a Restrictive Food Environment Intervention in a Rural Community Pharmacy Setting. *BMC Public Health.* 2016; 16:586) The study showed that people did not in fact go elsewhere to buy their pop. Sales showed a statistically insignificant drop in the town overall over the following nine months, relative to previous years. A small pharmacy that sold a mere 6% of the soda pop in town triggered a 17–32% overall drop in pop sales in the village when I removed this item from my shelves and shared with the public why I was doing it. This small victory for the health of my community reinforced in me the power a local pharmacy could have to educate. If you recall the types of studies we use in science, this was a "natural experiment," where subjects are exposed to a factor (withdrawal of sugary beverages) and a measurement was made (in this case the change in buying habits of sugary beverages). Everything else is out of control of the experimenters. The only variable measurement to determine was how far away from the village to take sales data.

The seasonal nature of the population of our village results in some widely variable sales during the course of the year. Even after controlling for this variability, it was interesting to see such a drop in sales. Statistically, the results were not found to be significant. Having said this, the authors of the study acknowledged that the results were clinically meaningful.

There didn't appear to be switching of where the pop was purchased after I discontinued selling it. The media coverage that the decision attracted probably played a role in this result, especially when one considers that my store sold pop as an "impulse buy," rather than serving the community as a primary destination for its purchase. Most importantly, I think that the decision generated a discussion within families about healthier eating habits. I do know that it inspired other pharmacy owners to reach out to me at the time and let me know of their plans to also take soft drinks off their shelves. More on this study in chapter 12.

Discontinuing the sugary beverages and bringing organic products into the store opened my eyes to a world of naysayers I was not previously aware of.

SUGAR

Please bear with me while I dive a little deeper into the history of our relationship with sugar. It is interesting that in 1972, a work called "Pure, White and Deadly" was published. It was written by John Yudkin, a British physiologist and nutritionist, and stated the dangers of the overconsumption of sugar. In it he concluded that not only cavities, but diabetes, obesity, cancer, and liver disease are all directly correlated with the amount of excess sugar consumed.

Yudkin's work was aggressively debunked by Ancel Keys, an American scientist who hypothesized after the "Seven Countries Study" that a "Mediterranean" style diet low in animal fat would result in lower heart disease incidence. Keys debated that there was absolutely no theoretical or experimental evidence to back up Yudkin's work.

When Yudkin passed away in 1995, his theories still had not made it into the mainstream of acceptance like they are today. His sugar theory has returned only in recent years in the *British Medical Journal.* As an interesting side note, both of these men lived into old age; however, Keys lived to the age of a hundred, whereas Yudkin died at (only) eighty-four.

Dr. David Ludwig showed us in a *Lancet* study in 2004 how high glycemic index carbs (fast-digesting, quick-absorption carbs) actually seemed to slow metabolism, increase fat storage, and raise triglyceride levels. They also disrupt the islet cells in the pancreas, which results in more insulin secretion than a diet with more low glycemic index carbs (slow-absorbing carbs). High glycemic index diets result in more overeating because they cause spikes in insulin and exacerbate hunger. (*Lancet.* 2004 Aug 28-Sep 3; 364 [9436]:778-85) It is important to note that the science of nutrition in weight gain is complex, and often needs more of an explanation than calories in and calories out.

THE ORGANIC FOOD STORY

When I stopped selling soda pop in my pharmacy, some people accused me of trying to control what they consume. More striking was the positive response from others when I began to sell organic food in response to a demand. As I have mentioned, I feel that people should try to reduce exposure to pro-inflammatory agents and avoid other "insults" that we discussed at the start of the chapter. Some argue that eating organic foods can theoretically be an efficient way to do this. There is no harm in trying to eat this way, but there is really nothing to back up the claim that nonorganic foods are harmful.

Why are people coming to my store asking for organic and non-GMO choices?

Several studies have backed up the correlation between exposure to pesticides and the incidence of Parkinson's disease, ALS, neurobehavioural performance, and dementia in the actual farmers and farmhands that use these toxins. (Kamel F, Hoppin JA. Association of pesticide exposure with Neurologic dysfunction and disease. *Environmental Health Perspectives.* 2004;112[9]) These pesticides include insecticides, herbicides, and fungicides. The best-documented health effects concerning occupational exposure of these chemicals involve the nervous system and neurodegenerative disease.

Insofar as consuming the food that has been treated with these chemicals, animal studies have shown a positive effect of an organic diet on weight, growth, fertility indices, and immune system function. (Huber, M. Metal. Organic food and impact on human health. *NJAS*. 58[3-4] pp 103-109L)

When I began to look at the effects of this type of exposure, I quickly realized that there are some very vocal individuals and groups out there. Eating organic foods is a way of eating that has many claims and a few benefits, but nonorganic isn't as bad as it is made out to be either.

GENETICALLY MODIFIED ORGANISMS

Increasingly, especially in Canada and the US, Genetically Modified Organisms (GMOs) have had their genetics altered so they express traits that humans consider to be beneficial. Plants that we eat are now often grown this way, most of the time without us realizing it, to make that food possess traits that are favourable to its growth – especially in a mass production environment. Genetically modifying an organism is about crop health, not necessarily about population health. Organisms can be altered to be more resistant to disease, pests, herbicides, salt, and drought, and to increase food supply. All of these benefits seem great; the issue some have is the unknown long-term health effects of human beings who consume these organisms.

The first use of genetically modified organisms was in 1980 when the US Supreme Court narrowly approved the first patent on a living organism, a bacteria that could eat up oil spills. Two years later, insulin appeared that was produced by E. coli bacteria, which was genetically engineered to make this crucial hormone. It would be a dozen more years before, in 1996, we saw our food altered by genetic engineering. The first GMO food-candidate presented for public acceptance was a slow-ripening tomato that lasted longer than conventional ones.

In this same year, genetically modified plants were approved for commercialization in Canada. In 1996, 1.7 million hectares worldwide were planted with GMO seeds. By 2009, there was an 80-fold increase to 134 million hectares, making GMOs the fastest growing crop technology in the world.

In present day, we are beginning to see nature recognizing our attempts to change genetics. We have seen bacteria developing resistance to antibacterial chemicals we have genetically introduced into our produce. We have also seen genetic traits being passed to other plants that were not genetically modified in the first place.

The issue here is that some feel we need long-term studies to really understand the effect of GMOs on our health. This is a time frame that is not realistic in comparison to the growth of the GMO industry and the strength of its lobby, so the experiment continues with real-time data. Given the short history GMOs have had on our planet, some people still feel we are lacking studies that back up its long-term safety.

The pro-GMO argument is that the GMO foods have not shown any adverse effects, so they are safe. This type of argument is known as the null hypothesis. Null hypothesis is part of the foundation on which both the scientific method and statistics are based. A null hypothesis means that there is no relationship between a determined cause and measured effect.

An example of a statistical analysis would be to measure the incidence of disease in one group who almost always eats non-GMO/ organic food and then to measure the incidence of disease in another group who almost always eats foods containing GMOs. If the incidence of disease appeared to be the same for both groups, then the hypothesis that GMOs cause disease would be "null" (or more correctly, not accepting the alternative hypothesis). Conversely, if we saw that people eating GMOs did have more diseases than our organic "control" group, we would say that we had found a "correlation," which would reject the null hypothesis.

Some arguments that are pro-GMO or anti-organic (though these two often coincide, it is important to note that they are not the same thing) state that we have not been able to statistically prove a cause-and-effect relationship between consuming GMO crops and any adverse health effects; therefore, there are no adverse effects, and any effect that is observed is by pure chance or a random event.

Conversely, the anti-GMO and pro-organic corners take the studies that have been done and use the ones showing a connection to further their argument. Hopefully, both sides have evaluated all studies to come to that conclusion. What makes it difficult for the general population is how two groups can arrive at the exact opposite conclusion after looking over the exact same data. Given the mistakes in the past on what we have been told is good for us and what is not, it is totally understandable to see a pushback from the assurance that nonorganic is a good thing.

Some of the genetically modified organisms created actually make compounds that act against herbicides so the crop can be sprayed with the herbicide and still survive, although the weeds die off. Geneticists have also created plants that can produce a pesticide to prevent insects from destroying them. One aspect of GMO foods often reported is the safety of the plant that we are eating, in that it can be grown without these harmful chemicals being applied to the growing plant in the field. (As a side note, I use the word "chemical" specifically because everything is a chemical, even water. Not all of them are bad.) To achieve these interesting outcomes, scientists are altering the DNA of the plants, so that the cells in the plants produce new proteins that can assemble the desired chemical compounds. There are a number of ways to do this, but one common way is to take DNA from another organism with a desired trait and splice that DNA into the DNA of your chosen plant. The problem with this and other genetic modification techniques is that we cannot be certain of the full effects of altering genetic information. We know the desired effect, but it is difficult to be certain that the desired effect is the only change that has occurred.

It is important to understand that short-term studies have shown results that seem to back both ways of growing and eating food – genetically or non-genetically modified. A 2011 study in the Eastern townships in the province of Quebec, Canada, investigated whether or not these herbicides or pesticides created by the crop are showing up in the bodies of pregnant women and their developing unborn babies. It was found that these compounds or their metabolites can be present in fetal blood and their mothers. This study helped direct the way for future studies on the effects of pesticides associated with genetically modified foods in maternal, fetal, and non-pregnant women's blood. One could argue that the pesticides and herbicides would still be present if the food were raised traditionally. It just saved the farmer from having to apply it. However, organically grown produce has significantly less of these products because they aren't applied to the crop.

(http://www.biosafety-info.net/bioart.php; https://www.uclm. es/Actividades/repositorio/pdf/doc_3721_4666.pdf)

It was later argued by a third party that the testing method done on the blood samples was not proven and may have been executed incorrectly. This was noted as a possible shortcoming in the text of the study.

In an effort to avoid bias based on individual studies, a systematic review was done which looked at twelve studies of longer than ninety days and twelve studies that involved two to five generations. This study concluded that GMO and non-GMO plants are nutritionally equivalent when used as food or feed. Small differences were observed but they were determined within statistical parameters to be insignificant. (http://www.sciencedirect.com/science/article/ pii/S0278691511006399)

PESTICIDES, HERBICIDES, AND FERTILIZERS

Not all nonorganic food is GMO. Some nonorganic food is standard produce which has been grown with the help of pesticides, herbicides, and fertilizers. What if you believe that genetically modified plants are of no consequence to your health, but you understand that added chemicals in your food is a bad idea?

Public concerns when chemicals like herbicides and pesticides are added to crops involve the potential for that chemical or its by-products to cause endocrine-disrupting effects, result in neurological development issues, or even cause increases in cancer.

Let's look at what science tells us about the use of fertilizers, pesticides, and other chemicals on crops. One systematic review of articles published between 1992 and 2003 found clear evidence in humans of neurologic outcomes, genotoxicity, and reproductive effects from pesticides (chemicals used to repel or kill insects, fungi, vegetation, and rodents). (http://www.ncbi.nlm.nih.gov/pmc/articles/PMC2231436/)

A common argument is the effect of herbicides, pesticides, and other chemicals on children. One such issue is childhood cancer, which has a mortality rate of 25% in Canada. Cancer-incidence graphs of all types can be misleading without knowing the background of the detection techniques that led to the statistics, the history of which treatment options became available when, or cultural factors such as smoking that influenced the incidence of cancer at various times. Hence, when we look at the steady increase in cancer from the late 1940s onward, it's easy to say that's when the advent of pesticide use really ramped up.

The Canadian Cancer Society states that the incidence of cancer is higher in farmers who apply pesticides to their crops. Farmers are obviously at a much higher exposure rate than the average person consuming the food. (http://

www.cancer.ca/en/prevention-and-screening/be-aware/
harmful-substances-and-environmental-risks/pesticides/?region=on)

So this not only becomes an issue of safety of the consumer, but also safety of the producer.

ORGANICS

If a food is labeled as 100% Organic or 100% Certified Organic, then it is generally free of genetically modified organisms. If you see wording such as "certified organic" or "made with organic," this means the food or product contains a small percentage of genetic modification.

In a large prospective study in the UK involving over 600,000 women, it was determined that there was no difference in cancer rates between women that never ate organic food as opposed to those who always ate organic food. (https://www.ncbi.nlm.nih.gov/pmc/articles/PMC4007233/) As much as I would like to connect the dots and lead someone to an obvious physiological pathway that eating organic is consistently superior to eating nonorganic foods, we just don't have that evidence in front of us right now. (https://www.sciencedirect.com/science/article/pii/S1573521411000054)

This is not to say that organic crops have no benefits. The levels of antioxidants have been shown to be higher in organic produce. (https://www.ncbi.nlm.nih.gov/pubmed/24968103) One reason for this is believed to be because antioxidant production is part of a mechanism by which plants stave off harm in lieu of pesticides. Also, vitamin C, zinc, and iron may be higher in organic produce.

In regard to any claim about cancer, nitrate levels have been found to be lower in organic food. The argument is that increased nitrates are correlated with higher incidence of cancer. (https://www.ncbi.nlm.nih.gov/pubmed/12002790)

Organic milk and meat have demonstrated higher levels of omega-3, which leads to less inflammation in the body. There has been found to be an inverse relationship between levels of omega-3 in the diet and telomere shortening on our chromosomes. Telomeres are the "end caps" that prevent deterioration of the chromosome. Shorter end caps means more susceptibility to damage in our DNA, with damaged DNA being associated with aging as well as age-related diseases. Oxidative stress is one of the main contributors to telomere shortening, another reason to consume antioxidant-rich organic foods.

Another reason for those recommending organic over nonorganic foods is the reduced levels of antibiotic residue on the organic plant. Reducing antibiotic exposure everywhere reduces the chance of antibiotic resistant organisms, a topic that may someday turn out to be our undoing, but which is beyond the scope of this book.

CONCLUDING THE DEBATE

My take on all of this is if you have a choice between one food that has been grown organically (hopefully in the true sense of the word) and one that has not, then you shouldn't stress out over consuming the one that is nonorganic. Again, I got rid of thirty-two feet of magazines and put in an organic section because I evaluated the validity of requests from my community. It turned out lots of people had been hoping for something like this in my little village. It was a huge hit and it blended well with what I was reinforcing in consultations anyway.

Personally, I don't think enough time has passed to determine all of the long-term effects of eating and growing genetically modified plants, but I can make an educated guess on what eating nonorganic food can do, based on what science has revealed thus far. My overall recommendations, based on my understanding of current research, are first based on what is safe for patients and second on what will most likely work for their overall well-being.

In contrast to the pro-organic argument, it is clear that we wouldn't be able to supply the food we do without the advances in GMO and the application of the chemicals we use to prevent disease in the plants. And we don't have any clear studies showing you will directly harm yourself by consuming these foods. But it's nice to have a choice. This brings us full circle to the notion that eating healthily is often a matter of socioeconomic privilege. Clearly, with food safety a concern for the planet and 20% of the population consuming 80% of the food resources (http://www.ncbi.nlm.nih.gov/pubmed/17457721), and with a growing overall population, this is our attempt at growing food in an economical way without consumers losing control of what they are eating. Regardless of whether you choose to eat organic or not, you still need a balanced diet – and by the way, you need exercise too.

FINAL THOUGHTS ON NUTRITION

Nutrition counselling is unfortunately not the strong point of a lot of healthcare professionals. Physicians, nurse practitioners, and pharmacists are in the perfect spot to counsel patients about their diet and also measure results and feedback on nutrition choices. However, your dietitian is your most important resource to make sense of the many "expert opinions" you hear. If you don't have access to a dietician, the simplest approach is to avoid trans fats and added sugars and eat a balanced diet without excess consumption. Skipping snacks between meals isn't a bad idea for most either. One thing I caution against is the growing trend of "organic snack food." Remember, wrapping a ribbon around a dying tree does nothing for the tree. Taking a snack food that is unhealthy and wrapping it in a ribbon of organic labels is no different, particularly if that food contains added sugar – natural or not. Organic food can also be processed.

The key is not to be miserable in your choices. If a particular choice leads to better health and makes you miserable, then it's time to find another way to be healthy. Lifestyles that attempt complete elimination of something that cannot be maintained will often result in a sense of failure. But if you are going to fall off the wagon and consume something unhealthy, make it the minimum amount that allows you to be happy.

If you are looking for a non-trendy way to eat for health, the Mediterranean diet has consistently delivered proven benefits. This diet promotes vegetables, fruits, nuts, seeds, legumes, potatoes, whole grains, breads, seafood, and extra virgin olive oil. There is some consumption of poultry, eggs, cheese, and yogurt, and very little red meat. The meal plan avoids added sugar, sugar-sweetened beverages, processed meat, refined grains, and processed foods. In other words, it's what common sense and growing consensus have been repeating for years.

Another diet often labelled as a fad, but from which I have seen impressive results, is the ketogenic diet. Caloric restriction and diets that are so low in carbohydrates they force the body to burn fat for fuel, also known as ketogenic diets, produce ketones in the body. This type of diet has been demonstrated in studies to help with autoimmune and autoinflammatory conditions like obesity, gout, diabetes, hypertension, asthma, psoriasis, and even MS and atherosclerosis. More study is needed in ketogenic recommendations with regard to specific diseases before a widespread recommendation can be given.

It is important to note that there is no one ideal diet that works for every single person, especially for weight loss. Beware of claims that lead you into believing that one diet is "the best" for losing weight over all others. I have seen people struggle with weight loss that took a toll on them mentally because of results that didn't meet expectations. A healthy weight is one that doesn't necessarily rely on a scale for happiness. The healthiest weight you can maintain at an enjoyable level is what you should strive for.

On the other hand, I have seen people following the ketogenic diet come off their medications for asthma, arthritis, cholesterol, and high blood pressure, as well as all of their insulin doses – no more insulin. Now, you can argue that any weight loss could do this, but one patient actually came off all of those medications. It was the most extreme case I had seen in twenty-four years. I have heard from many of my customers that ketogenic diets can improve sleep as well, which incidentally, is where we turn next.

CHAPTER 3

SLEEP

"The last refuge of the insomniac
is a sense of superiority to
the sleeping world."

– LEONARD COHEN

Sleep is one of the most important and least understood factors contributing to our overall well-being. In fact, health outcomes as diverse as cardiovascular problems, insulin resistance, anxiety, alcohol misuse, and overall mortality can all be linked to decreased sleep.

In this chapter we will examine some of the mechanics behind sleep. We will discuss some common sleep disorders and sleep-related diseases. Finally, we will talk about ways to improve our sleep, first, using pharmaceuticals, and second, by improving our overall sleep hygiene.

THE SLEEP CYCLE

Sleep can be broken down into different phases that reflect how deep you are into the sleep pattern. In a normal, healthy sleep pattern, these stages go from phases one to four and then rapid eye movement (REM) sleep. This will typically cycle over 90-minute periods during the night, with REM sleep occurring for longer periods as morning approaches. In this way, your sleep gets deeper as the night progresses – hopefully. Phase one is very light sleep. In fact, most people brought out of phase one would argue that they really weren't asleep at all. Sound familiar? This phase is also where you might experience the annoying but harmless sudden jerking or falling motion that wakes you.

This is followed by the second phase of light sleep, phase two, where there is a further slowing of brain waves. In phase three, we see a growing pattern of delta waves in the brain activity, and deep sleep is initiated. If someone wakes you and it takes half an hour to get back to normal, you were at least in phase three. In phase four, we see delta waves in the brain almost exclusively. Although muscle activity and eye movement are mostly gone in these last two deepest forms of sleep, this is where we experience night terrors, sleepwalking, and bed-wetting.

The fifth stage of sleep, called REM (rapid eye movement), shows a vastly different brain wave pattern. It might even appear that the person is awake because of the amount of brain wave activity. Your muscles are completely relaxed in phase four, but they become for the most part paralyzed in REM sleep, which could be a protective mechanism to prevent you from harming yourself during this active form of sleep.

THE SLEEP-WAKE CYCLE

Sleep is regulated by a function of your circadian rhythm known as the sleep-wake cycle. The circadian rhythm is an internal 24-hour clock that uses hormones and neural activity to regulate functions throughout the body. As a general rule, maintaining a consistent circadian rhythm by eating and going to sleep at regular times every day is essential for good health. The sleep-wake cycle is a function of your circadian rhythm that heavily relies on two hormones: melatonin and cortisol.

Melatonin is a hormone that the pineal gland produces from an amino acid called tryptophan. It is a key chemical ingredient in creating the sensation of sleepiness. The more melatonin you have in your system, the sleepier you will feel. The pineal gland's production of melatonin is influenced by the presence of light. The more light that you are exposed to, the less melatonin you will produce. We will discuss problems with melatonin regulation in greater detail later in this chapter.

Cortisol is a hormone secreted by the adrenal gland at various intervals throughout the day. Cortisol is commonly recognized by most people as the "fight or flight" chemical, because it is released in large amounts during stressful situations. In fact, cortisol plays an important role in regulating most human behaviour. In a normal day, where nothing particularly traumatic happens, cortisol levels begin to rise as part of the body's waking process. Levels reach their highest points around breakfast time and slowly descend in peaks and valleys that align roughly with mealtimes until it's time for bed. At bedtime, cortisol levels should be the lowest they have been all day. As you may guess, this corresponds with a feeling of calmness which, in combination with rising levels of melatonin, should result in a good night's sleep.

Unfortunately, for many people this just is not the case.

It is common to hear from patients in the pharmacy that they just can't seem to turn their brains off at night. This sometimes requires more than just a sedating agent and can require a deeper look into what prevents your brain from reaching sleep. Being sleep-deprived for just one night has been shown to increase your body's cortisol levels the following night. If this negative process gets out of hand, this is one way we can end up with the problem known as insomnia.

Sleep loss results in an elevation of cortisol levels the next evening. (Leproult R1, Copinschi G, Buxton O, Van Cauter E. Sleep loss results in an elevation of cortisol levels the next evening. *Sleep*. 1997 Oct;20[10]:865-70)

INSOMNIA

The most common sleep problem that I receive inquiries about at the pharmacy is insomnia. Insomnia may be defined as a difficulty initiating sleep, maintaining sleep (frequent awakenings or trouble returning to sleep after these awakenings) and early morning wakening with an inability to fall back asleep. (John W. Winkelman, M.D., Ph.D. Insomnia Disorder. *N Engl J Med* 2015; 373:1437-1444 October 8, 2015. DOI: 10.1056/NEJMcp1412740)

Insomnia correlates strongly with depression, diabetes, acute myocardial infarction, heart failure, hypertension, and coronary artery disease.

Although we know that insomnia is a common symptom in psychiatric problems (Seow E, Seng L, et al, Identifying the Best Sleep Measure to Screen Clinical Insomnia in a Psychiatric Population, *Sleep Medicine*, Volume 0, Issue 0). Like generalized anxiety disorder, randomized trials are lacking to show any specific and recommendable benefits of sleep hygiene in preventing or improving this disorder.

Depression and insomnia are so linked that insomnia is used as an indicator of depression. As with anxiety, insomnia may be a separate condition that runs independent of depression, even though they often occur together. One thing is for certain: diet, exercise, and sleep all have some role in the development, progression, and treatment of depression. (Lopresti AL, Hood SD, Drummond PD. A review of lifestyle factors that contribute to important pathways associated with major depression: diet, sleep and exercise. *J Affect Disord.* 2013 May 15;148[1]:12-27. DOI: 10.1016/j.jad.2013.01.014. Epub 2013 Feb 14.)

WOMEN AND SLEEP

We also know insomnia strikes women more than men and is also more common in shift workers, who are also more likely to suffer from ulcers, obesity, cancer, hypercholesterolemia, diabetes, metabolic disease, and depression. (Céline Vetter, PhD, et al. Association Between Rotating Night Shift Work and Risk of Coronary Heart Disease Among Women. *JAMA.* 2016;315[16]:1726-1734. DOI:10.1001/jama.2016.4454) I am often asked about the topic of "sleep hygiene," or the correct way to sleep, and have presented this topic on a number of occasions to the public and to work groups. It is especially disheartening to tell a room full of shift-working nurses that they are more susceptible to all of the problems I listed above, when they are the ones helping others' medical issues.

While many issues can affect women's sleep, menopause is easily one of the top reasons patients come to us for decreased sleep quality. As we will see later, treatment options for this biologically normal yet annoying event can aid in dramatically improving sleep quality and quantity. As estrogen declines, we see an increase in hot flashes and a loss of sleep due to hot flashes. The fluctuating nature of estrogen levels as they gradually decline doesn't help when the body tries to deal with one level one minute and another level the next. Cortisol levels also tie in with hot flashes as they do with sleep. Women often claim a hot flash ties in with a cortisol-raising event like a stressful incident or a bout of hunger.

Hormone replacement therapy (HRT) will often help with these symptoms. However, I have found it increasingly difficult to find prescribers for any type of HRT since a study came out in early 2000s, The Women's Health Initiative Study, which sought to determine the effect of hormones in menopause and how they relate to disease. Unfortunately, the error was in the takeaway that HRT contributed to breast cancer and heart attacks. As a result, an entire generation of women were for the most part left to fend for themselves with their suffering of menopause symptoms. It turned out the study was stopped abruptly because the authors claimed an increase in breast cancer and heart attacks, when in fact there were not statistically significant findings for either. An increase in venous clots and a reduction in hip fractures were the only statistically significant findings.

As a result, women found themselves with countless sleepless nights as well as unnecessary harm and early death as their hormones dropped to that of men their age. That is a topic for another day, but prescribing habits never returned to normal, and pharmacies that reached out to help these women were often left empty-handed and trying to explain the difference between a progestin and progesterone.

RESTLESS LEG SYNDROME

Restless leg syndrome is another disorder that can have those afflicted at their wits' end as to what to do. There is certainly no shortage of prescription drugs that try to help with this affliction. I have witnessed treatments that work with some with success, but no one treatment works for everyone.

Non-prescription supplements may help, but only for those with suboptimal iron levels (*Sleep Med.* 2013 Nov;14[11]:1100-4. DOI: 10.1016/j.sleep.2013.06.006. Epub 2013 Aug 28). Low iron is *not* a condition you want to treat through guesswork. If you think you might be low on iron, get your iron levels tested.

One small study found vitamin D helpful in treating restless legs. It appears that the average vitamin D blood concentration was low in the study subjects, but when the vitamin D blood levels came back up with supplementation, the symptoms of restless leg syndrome decreased. Patients with normal levels of this vitamin should expect very little effect. (Wali S, Shukr A, Boudal A, et al. *Sleep Breath* [2015] 19: 579. DOI: https://doi.org/10.1007/s11325-014-1049-y)

Calcium and magnesium, two elements that are commonly low, have been shown to help with restless legs but with unconvincing and mixed clinical results published over the years. In my pharmacy however, I have witnessed positive results with both compounds. Calcium and magnesium also have the advantage of being inexpensive, and most people are in need of supplementing them anyway. Given their relatively safe side-effect profile, it is worth a short trial on either calcium or magnesium supplements to gauge a response. However, a common class of blood-pressure medications called calcium channel blockers can exacerbate restless legs.

Other supplements like B vitamins, especially folate, have also been tried with a little more research to back up the correlation between low folate and restless legs, especially in pregnancy. Folic acid is a supplement I recommend in low amounts only, under 400 mcg daily. Levels of 400 mcg to 1000 mcg daily should be taken only under the supervision of your healthcare practitioner.

SLEEP AND WEIGHT GAIN

There has been some speculation that there is a causal relationship between poor sleep and weight gain. As of now, the picture is less clear with adults than with children. Short sleep duration correlates positively with weight gain in children. (Magee, Lorrie et al. Longitudinal associations between sleep duration and subsequent weight gain: A systematic review. *Sleep Medicine Reviews*, Volume 16, Issue 3, 231-241) Some studies seem to show that a shorter sleep duration is associated with a modest increase in future weight gain in adults, but their results are less substantial. (Sanjay R. Patel, Atul Malhotra, David P. White, Daniel J. Gottlieb, and Frank B. Hu. Association between Reduced Sleep and Weight Gain in Women. Sleep Hygiene *Am. J. Epidemiol.* [15 November 2006] 164 [10]: 947-954)

The association in adults between sleep duration and obesity is a complex one. At least we know that lack of sleep does not appear to cause one to reduce weight. As one weight-loss customer told me, "You can't expect to stay up late every night and not get hungry and start to eat." This candid statement rings true for many people.

SLEEP AND DISEASE

Here, we discuss sleep deprivation and its effects on insulin sensitivity and cortisol secretion. Type 2 diabetes is a disease where the body develops a resistance to the effect of insulin. Type 2 diabetes has also been associated with amount of sleep, in that each one makes the other worse. (Barone, Mark TU et al. Diabetes and sleep: A complex cause-and-effect relationship. *Diabetes Research and Clinical Practice.* Volume 91, Issue 2, 129-137)

Too little or too much sleep correlates with a higher incidence of type 2 diabetes. Between seven and eight hours seems to be the sweet spot for how long the average adult needs to sleep. Insulin sensitivity seems to be related to sleep because of sleep's emerging relationship with inflammation. Let's dig deeper.

Inflammatory markers seem to be influenced by amount of sleep; because of this connection, many seemingly unassociated conditions may be more connected than we thought. Studies have found that lack of sleep increases inflammatory markers in the blood, and that this inflammation may perpetuate lack of sleep.

Increase in inflammatory markers leads to metabolic stress, which in turn leads to insulin resistance as a defense mechanism. Insulin resistance correlates with an increase in all-cause mortality, which includes heavy hitters like cardiovascular disease and, of course, type 2 diabetes.

An increase in the amount of insulin in the blood, known as hyperinsulinemia, resulting from insulin resistance, is one of our number one agers. Increased insulin levels also cause retinal vessel damage, which is related to brain atrophy and dementia, even in non-diabetic individuals. Insulin levels also increase with obesity, as do triglycerides as the HDL good cholesterol decreases.

While all of this does not mean that lack of sleep directly causes dementia, obesity, depression, anxiety, diabetes, heart disease, a bad lipid profile, or inflammation, it is interesting to note the very close relationship among all of them. Statistically, the common denominator is sleep.

SLEEP DEPRIVATION AND GENERAL HEALTH

While the effects of sleep deprivation on your overall health can be difficult to measure, there are ways the scientific community has attempted to do so. The most direct cause-and-effect sleep-deprivation studies are where study subjects are prevented from sleeping, and scientists measure the effects on the patients. In a systematic review of such studies, it was found that increased blood pressure correlated positively with lack of sleep. In fact, it has been found that just one night of sleep deprivation can result in increased blood pressure the entire next day.

In a large study involving over 30,000 subjects, sleep question-naires were used to determine sleep quality and duration. The study then compared these factors to disease states and markers like body mass index, obesity, hypertension, cholesterol levels, diabetes, stroke, and heart attack. This study found that both sleep insufficiency and duration are related to cardiometabolic health. To add to the growing pile of information as to why sleep deprivation is not good for you, meta-analyses on a number of studies have been done to confirm the effects of too much or too little sleep on all causes of mortality. These analyses found that less than seven or more than eight hours of sleep per day resulted in a higher mortality rate and also an increased risk of coronary heart disease and stroke. (Ferrie, JE. et al. Sleep Epidemiology – a Rapidly Growing Field. *International Journal of Epidemiology.* 40.6 [2011]: 1431-1437. PMC. Web. 30 Apr. 2016) Achieving the optimal amount of sleep is certainly a fine line to walk.

Of course, these types of studies are not the direct observational cause-and-effect sleep studies mentioned earlier. Instead, we look more at trends of self-reported sleep duration and life expectancy and disease. Any study that bases its data on recall, be it diet, sleep, or exercise, is at the mercy of the subjective brain recalling the event. Recall is unreliable enough when we are awake. While this doesn't result in an iron-clad cause-and-effect correlation, the repeated results on these types of studies have led to the sleep recommendations we have today.

One thing that has grown from this collection of data is that, aside from diet and exercise, sleep quality is a third critical compo-nent in the promotion of a healthy lifespan. The inflammatory response to too much or too little sleep is now recognized and cannot be ignored. C-reactive protein (CRP) and interleukin 6 (IL-6) levels are increased with longer than eight hours' sleep duration as well as with insomnia and shorter durations of sleep. (Irwin, MR. et al. Sleep Disturbance, Sleep Duration, and Inflammation: A Systematic Review and Meta-Analysis of Cohort Studies and Experimental Sleep Deprivation. *Biological Psychiatry*. Volume 80, Issue 1, 40-52.)

Sleep is truly a regenerative and restorative part of our lives. You may not be interested in applying animal studies directly to humans, but you might be interested in knowing that rats that are consistently deprived of REM sleep live shorter lives than those that experience REM sleep regularly.

ANXIETY

I want to talk about anxiety because I often observe poor sleep and anxiety to be related in the patients that come into my pharmacy. What is a doctor or a pharmacist to do when presented with a patient with a complaint of anxiety? If we are going to choose the route of medication, my first concern is always that we find something evidence-based and safe. If Relora isn't something you've heard of, I recommend taking some time to learn about it, especially if "nonaddictive" and "nonsedating" are words that are as important to you as they are to me. Although there aren't extensive studies to rely on, one good, randomized, placebo-controlled, double-blind trial has shown promise with reduction in anxiety with minimal sedation. (Talbott, SM, Talbott JA, Pugh M. Effect of Magnolia Officinalis and Philodendron Amurense [Relora®] on Cortisol and Psychological Mood State in Moderately Stressed Subjects. *Journal of the International Society of Sports Nutrition*. 10 [2013]: 37. PMC. Web. 1 May 2016)

Critics will quickly point out that the problem with this study is that it was sponsored by the manufacturer of Relora at the time.

This type of conflict of interest is a double-edged sword, because although double-blind studies are demanded by many skeptics of supplements, these same skeptics feel that the results can almost be nullified if the company paying for the trial is also manufacturing the product. But if we are pushing companies to back up what they are selling, this type of evidence is better than no evidence. Also, most prescription drugs have their studies done by the company that sells them. In my experience, this product is worth trying first over prescription medications.

However, if anxiety is getting the best of you despite trying non-prescription options, it is also my opinion that several prescription medications are absolutely amazing when used correctly for anxiety. Typically, the older antihistamines and older antidepressants are more sedating but not recommended for the elderly (who need it the most). Some newer antidepressants like Sertraline are good for anxiety without being as sedating in comparison. In any case, solving one's anxiety can be a key to getting to sleep.

SLEEPING PILLS

Sleeping pills are marketed as being useful in the short term, but most of the patients I see are on these medications for life. It is for this reason that I am not a huge fan of one of the biggest classes of prescriptions that I fill daily. Sleeping pills have been implicated in memory issues and even associated with worsening dementia. Apart from the REM-suppressing effects of these drugs, they also suppress stages three and four of sleep. They keep you sleeping longer, but in a lighter form of sleep. It's no wonder that those on sleeping pills often experience drowsiness and confusion. In fact, long-term patients on sleeping pills have such deep-sleep deprivation and lack of REM sleep that they often begin to experience anxiety which, again, is part of the reason they may have been put on them in the first place. For this reason, sleeping pills should only be prescribed for short-term or sporadic use. However, if sleeping pills are something your physician has determined through risk-benefit analysis will work for you, do not stop them just because of the opinion you have read here. Consult your physician before making any changes to an existing prescription plan.

Despite the possibility of negative side effects, some sleeping pills help you. The sedative properties of antihistamine medications are sought after for their sleeping-pill effects, but unfortunately their effect on sleep architecture, namely their effect on REM sleep reduction, is a major drawback. Doxepin, an antidepressant at doses starting at 25 mg, affects mainly histamine receptors at 1, 3, and 6 mg and seems to affect sleep architecture much less. It has become a growing popular option even for seniors based on its low side-effect profile and lack of abuse or withdrawal issues.

A fair number of prescriptions for sleeping pills involve the benzodiazepines described below.

BENZODIAZEPINES

As a pharmacist, I often see a group of drugs called benzodiazepines used for sleep. This common and old group of prescription drugs does work to put you to sleep and hopefully keep you there, if that is your only goal. The issue with these medications is that they are known suppressors of phases three and four sleep and of the coveted REM sleep, during which the brain organizes thoughts; allows you to better recall events, facts, and details; releases growth hormones; and synthesizes proteins.

Children and young adults experience more phase three and four sleep than older adults do. In fact, most elderly people sleep only in phases one and two. This is why, in my opinion, younger adults may be more prone to the long-term side effects of sleeping pills. You will remember that sleeping pills inhibit phase three and four sleep in favour of more phase two sleep, which is not as restful. In older people, the use of the benzodiazepine group of sleeping pills is more justifiable. In a demographic that is physiologically expecting a deep phase of sleep, inhibiting this sleep could mean negative effects for memory consolidation and information processing, despite the fact that there may be some of this partially taking place in phase two sleep as well. It should be noted here that the effects that these medications have on disruption of sleep architecture are largely speculative. We just know that the type of sleep normally seen in humans is affected, especially sleep that we understand to be restorative. The effects these medications have on memory and psychological conditions, as well as negative effects on long-term health, are still open for study.

An interesting hormonal depletion that happens because of the benzodiazepines is with melatonin. Many patients have told me how they have tried to come off these medications used either for anxiety or sleep and have insomnia to some degree. You will recall that melatonin is key in regulating our sleep-wake cycle, and with the sedative taken away it can be difficult to sleep, unless the medication is withdrawn gradually. Supplementing with melatonin can help with this. In a 1999 study in Tel Aviv, it was found that of thirty-four elderly patients who were coming off their benzodiazepines and divided into two groups, the ones that took a melatonin supplement (in this case, 2 mg, long-acting, within two hours of bedtime) were 78% more successful in reducing their benzodiazepine use by five or six weeks. In comparison, in the placebo group, only 25% had successfully come off the sleeping pill by week six. (Garfinkel, Doron, et al. Facilitation of benzodiazepine discontinuation by melatonin. *Archives of Internal Medicine*, Vol. 159, November 8, 1999, pp. 2456-60)

MELATONIN

A discussion of sleep issues wouldn't be complete without mentioning melatonin. We have already spoken about melatonin as a hormone created by the pineal gland, but we have also been able to synthesize melatonin as a supplement. As with many medical problems, it is often interesting, if not productive, to look for a deficiency that is causing the problem in the first place. This is where melatonin comes in. Symptoms of low melatonin include restless legs, tense muscles, fatigue, anxious thinking on wakening, seasonal affective disorder, irritability, abdominal pain, and increased intestinal spasms. It is also proposed that those with low melatonin correlate with many disease states, such as high blood pressure, heart disease, obesity, diabetes, Alzheimer's disease, and certain cancers.

I suppose one way to find out if you have a deficiency in melatonin is to try it and see if it works. This approach is not overly scientific but, aside from possible grogginess the next day, melatonin has very few known negative side effects, so it is safe to experiment with if sleep is an issue for you. Doses are typically 3-6 mg, although some patients will not respond until they get to 15 mg or more. The truth is that melatonin does help certain individuals sleep and is completely useless in others. It depends if your sleep problem is actually stemming from a lack of hormonal melatonin.

If you are deficient in melatonin, taking a melatonin pill a couple of hours before bedtime may help you fall asleep. I have also seen patients who tend to wake up during the night respond well to a melatonin dose right at bedtime.

You can help your own body's melatonin levels by exposing yourself to light when you get up and removing that light when you go to bed. We will talk in greater detail about the issue of screen time at the end of this chapter. While studies on these phenomena are slim, it appears that red and amber light do not affect melatonin production, but blue, green, and white lights do. Holding most smart phones twelve inches from your face at the highest light setting seems to limit alterations to melatonin production while anywhere closer will lower melatonin levels. This recommendation changes, however, when we are talking about a tablet-sized screen, a regular laptop computer screen, or a television.

OVER-THE-COUNTER MEDS FOR SLEEP

Valerian

I am often asked about valerian for sleep. Many sleep studies about supplements and herbs do not include a placebo group to compare results, making these studies susceptible to the placebo effect. For example, the act of taking a pill may cause drowsiness if a subject believes that is the pill's purpose.

To try to get into the various studies of valerian can be futile, since valerian includes 200 different species and is prepared with different extraction techniques among so many different brands on the shelf. There are also different compounds found in valerian products, so inconsistent results are not all that uncommon. This is a common problem with herbal preparations. The scientific community is not clear on which compound in the valerian is actually at work in sleep promotion. It also appears to be an unstable compound if not packaged in a timely manner. Studies on valerian can be difficult to compare; some studies are favourable, and others are unfavourable in finding valerian useful for sleep. Aside from showing inconsistent results, many of the studies are small in subject enrollment, making it difficult to determine the actual effect of the supplement over random results.

My opinion on this over-the-counter sleep aid is that valerian is certainly safe to try. You often get what you pay for with supplements, so keep that in mind when you see 1000 tablets for $1.99. Valerian tends to work better with continuous use rather than as needed. An interesting note is that valerian has been compared to the benzodiazepine prescriptions for sleep, with comparable results between the two in reducing time to get to sleep and less daytime sedation. Withdrawal can occur just like the benzodiazepines though, if abruptly stopped. Although valerian shouldn't make you drowsy in the morning, it can for a few hours after taking it, so keep this in mind if you are planning to do something that requires alertness.

Other Natural Sleep Aids

Other natural products we see used for sleep are lemon balm, kava, hops, passionflower, skullcap, and casein hydrolysate, all with inconsistent results. Again, as with any OTC aid, especially one in the supplement or herb section, it is imperative that you check with your pharmacist before buying.

Theanine is another favourite of mine for relaxation and sleep. Theanine is found in abundance in the leaves of green tea. Drinking the tea isn't applicable here but rather just the supplement. It is found in two forms, d-theanine and l-theanine. These two forms are quite different in their actions. The l- form is absorbed at three times the rate of the d- form. It is for this reason that most forms we see on sale are l-theanine. Taking a combination of the two isn't helpful, as the d- form prevents the l- form from being absorbed. The neurotransmitters dopamine and serotonin are both increased with the presence of l-theanine (Yokogoshi H, Mochizuki M, Saitoh K. Theanine induced reduction of brain serotonin concentration in rats. *Biosci Biotech Biochem.* 62 [4] 1998; 816-17), and l-theanine also causes relaxation and improves sleep.

Similarly, **5-HTP** is another sought-after supplement for sleep. Otherwise known as L-5-hydroxytryptophan, it is the precursor to the neurotransmitter serotonin. Although its effectiveness in treating depression by targeting this neurotransmitter may be a bit exaggerated (personally I do not recommend it at all), its use in sleep disorders is more founded. It has been tested with positive results for night terrors in children. (Bruni O1, Ferri R, Miano S, Verrillo E. L -5-Hydroxytryptophan treatment of sleep terrors in children. *Eur J Pediatr.* 2004 Jul;163[7]:402-7. Epub 2004 May 14) Despite very few studies showing the effectiveness of 5-HTP in sleep, I find that it works for some people, although it can take from six to twelve weeks to do so. However, due to its side-effect profile and interaction potential with other meds, it isn't something that I recommend lightly.

Controlling the effect of cortisol can also affect sleep. Not only a high level of cortisol but also a low level of cortisol can impair sleep, even though you feel fatigued. In some people, exercise near bedtime can inhibit sleep because it raises cortisol too much; while in others, exercise can bring the cortisol up to normal levels and allow for sleep. Optimal cortisol levels can also be maintained by avoiding alcohol, smoking, caffeine, sugar, bread, pasta, and cereal. Coincidentally, these are the things we have already discussed avoiding before bed in order to get a good night's sleep. These sugary items increase insulin, which in turn lowers cortisol in the short term. Hormones are very interconnected in their effects.

What else lowers your cortisol levels? Evidence points to a few things that can help. Phosphatidylserine is commonly touted as a cortisol lowering agent. Although held back by small study sizes with a relatively low number of human patients, results do show the cortisol-blunting effect of this molecule. (Starks MA, Starks SL, Kingsley M, Purpura M, Jäger R. The effects of phosphatidylserine on endocrine response to moderate intensity exercise. *Journal of the International Society of Sports Nutrition.* 2008; 5:11. DOI:10.1186/1550-2783-5-11) So far, evidence isn't stellar, but for most people, the supplement is safe to try short-term if you are looking for an alternative to a prescription sleeping pill.

ACUPUNCTURE AND TRADITIONAL MEDICINE

I have received many anecdotal reports from my patients who have sought out acupuncture to improve sleep. As always, my belief is that if you are happy with the results, then go ahead. Studies on acupuncture are often flawed in some way, either in study design, lack of follow-up, or small sample size. A Cochrane review looked at seven English trials and concluded that there was no benefit to acupuncture in relation to sleep. Cochrane is notoriously conservative in its recommendations, but a Chinese review of six studies came to the same conclusion. Another review of 46 randomized trials concluded that acupuncture increases sleep duration and quality, but admitted that many shortcomings were observed in the trials it surveyed. (Cao, Huijuan et al. Acupuncture for Treatment of Insomnia: A Systematic Review of Randomized Controlled Trials. *Journal of Alternative and Complementary Medicine.* 15.11 (2009): 1171-86. PMC. Web. 12 May 2016)

Do I recommend acupuncture for sleep? Based on the evidence, no, but if you are at the end of your rope and it won't put you in the poorhouse, go ahead and give it a try. I realize this is not a glowing endorsement, but as always, my first priority is safety, followed by effectiveness. Just don't sell the farm in order to try it.

SLEEP HYGIENE

We have discussed various pharmaceutical solutions that may help you improve your sleep. Before you pursue any of these avenues, I advise you to take some time to see if fixing your sleep hygiene can improve your slumber. Of course, the best approach to dealing with lack of sleep is to address any primary issues. If there is pain or an underlying mood disorder, then address those first. If the room is too noisy, too hot, cold, too uncomfortable, too bright, or whatever, deal with that.

Practice good sleep hygiene by following simple steps. You should have a regular wind-down ritual before going to bed. When you enter your bedroom, your mind should automatically switch to a sleep mode. You should do everything you can to make this transition simple or even subconscious. This wind-down ritual can involve no reading in bed, no TV in the bedroom, no music in the bedroom, no pets in the bedroom, no extremes of heat or cold, no lights, nothing that will give the brain a chance to derail from proceeding to sleep.

It is important to preserve your sleep environment as much as possible. This means no light from your window or from a computer, phone screen, nightlight, or clock radio. Everything must be removed that emits light or blocked from emitting light. Light-blocking eye shields may be more practical.

Also, if you are still awake after fifteen or twenty minutes, it's best to get out of bed. This indicates that your brain has not engaged its sleep gear, so to speak. At this point, you need to reset your mind's software by leaving the bedroom (or bed, if it is a one-room apartment) and sit out in the living room on your couch for a bit. You can casually flip through a magazine (nothing that will engage your mind too much) and then return to bed when you begin to feel sleepy.

It is also important to go to bed and to wake up at roughly the same times every day, weekends included. If you did not sleep well last night, don't try to make up for it by sleeping during the day (sleeping in that morning or going to bed early the next evening). Stick to your guns and maintain those same hours. A short nap (twenty minutes) in the afternoon is permitted to refresh your mind, but that is it.

Sleep hygiene discourages the concept of the afternoon nap for the most part, although a short nap can sometimes be beneficial. Nap philosophy differs all over the world and among age groups, but there does appear to be some benefit. Most of us have experienced the fatigue involved with driving a car for too long. In fact, more car accidents occur from nodding off (also known as micro-sleeping) at around two p.m. than at six p.m. This type of nodding off is common with many medications that are given for reasons other than stress or sleep. Having a nap that is short enough that you awaken before phase three sleep is beneficial because it avoids the sleep inertia that can follow deep sleep. Learning and recall have also been shown to markedly improve with these short fifteen-to-twenty-minute naps during the day.

It's best not to eat anything at least three hours before bedtime. Too many refined carbs in the evening, especially without the blunting effect of fibre, can result in a spike of insulin that causes a dive in your blood glucose in the middle of the night. This will cause a cortisol release to regain your sugar levels. This hormone causes you to wake up if secreted in too high a level. Especially important to avoid are snacks with refined carbs and high glycemic index foods like white bread, desserts, potatoes, rice, most breakfast cereals, and dried fruit with little or no fibre or protein to slow the sugar absorption down.

Also, avoid caffeine after twelve noon (some of us are very slow metabolizers of caffeine – if you don't know whether or not you are, just assume you are). No nicotine in the evening is often recommended, but it isn't clear if this has any effect, especially if withdrawal starts to kick in at bedtime. It is clear that smokers typically have more insomnia than nonsmokers.

Alcohol abstinence in the evening is recommended for similar reasons, as people suffering from insomnia also tend to drink more and closer to bedtime. Alcohol consumption typically results in the patient falling asleep better but consistently waking more frequently during the night as the alcohol is metabolized and removed from the body. As well, the diuretic effect of alcohol increases urination during the night. Increased apnea, snoring, and disrupted sleep structure are all problems associated with alcohol. Alcohol consumption near bedtime diminishes deep sleep.

There is also the issue of what alcohol does to blood sugar during the middle of the night when consumed before bedtime. Low blood sugar spikes cortisol, which is released from your adrenal glands in a protective effort to prevent hypoglycemia, which wakes you up – another reason to avoid eating and drinking before bed.

Studies have shown that consistent adherence to proper sleep hygiene techniques results in better overall sleep and sleep quality for people of all ages. (Mindell, Jodi A. et al. Developmental aspects of sleep hygiene: Findings from the 2004 National Sleep Foundation Sleep in America Poll. *Sleep Medicine.* Volume 10, Issue 7, 771-79). Repeated studies show that certain habits and activities such as those mentioned above should be avoided in order to improve sleep. (Jefferson et al. Sleep Hygiene and Insomnia. *Sleep.* Vol. 28, No. 5, 2005)

Studies that compare sleep hygiene to a control group with no intervention are difficult to find. This puts most of these recommendations into the realm of common sense rather than "evidence-based." Rigorous improvement of sleep hygiene has never been proven to be more helpful than the standard proven therapies of the common benzodiazepines and the non-benzodiazepine sedatives, or antidepressants, for sleep. One thing is for sure, the phases of sleep that reflect a deeper sleep are reached with better sleep hygiene and are often not achieved with prescription or over-the-counter medicine. As we get older, the list of meds we should avoid increases (the Beers list) because our bodies are affected by side effects in a more pronounced manner, like unsteadiness that may cause a fall. This cuts down on sleep options available to us as we age.

SLEEP AND SMARTPHONES

Above all, when you are going to bed, no phones! The growing belief that we have disrupted sleep when we have more screen time near (or after) bedtime has not gone unseen by the companies that make these products. These companies have begun talking like neuroscientists in the hope of keeping us on our smartphones well after we have gone to bed. I know that I am guilty of this.

The shift from blue light to red light on smartphone screens is an attempt to soften the bad rep smartphones and tablets have in order to keep us dependent on them as many hours as possible in a twenty-four-hour day. What we need to understand is that all light increases alertness and affects the body's natural clock and our ability to have a quality sleep.

For the entire length of human history, humans have been communicating in the same way, only to be abruptly disrupted within an incredibly short ten-year time span by the smartphone. It is still far too early to make conclusions about the effects that this massive technological change will have on our sleep patterns and across all other aspects of our lives. It is now estimated that we get, on average, eighteen fewer minutes of sleep per night than our parents did. Most of this is due to the 24/7 nature of our lifestyles. As a father of four boys, I absolutely see differences in sleep habits between them and myself growing up. A notable offender involves excessive smartphone and tablet use.

The evidence is clear: the less stimulation of the brain, the better the sleep. Virtually across all types of screens, sleep time suffers with more exposure. (Hale, L, Guan, S. Screen time and sleep among school-aged children and adolescents: a systematic literature review. *Sleep Med Review.* 2015 Jun; 21:50-8) Screen time in a developing brain has shown adverse effects even while the child is awake during the day. So, in conclusion, an hour before bed, if you can, if you are strong enough, turn off your phone! Your body will thank you. Moderation is best.

One final habit that has been scientifically proven to improve sleep is exercise. No matter how old you are or what state your body is in, you can almost always benefit from a good workout. Let's find out more about exercise in Chapter 4.

CHAPTER 4

EXERCISE

"My grandmother started walking five miles a day when she was sixty. She's ninety-seven now, and we don't know where the heck she is."

– ELLEN DEGENERES

Nutrition and sleep are essential topics in any discussion on well-being and longevity. Without talking about exercise, there would be a huge missing link. Let's get right to the most commonly argued point in the topic of exercise: the debate as to what exercise really does for us. I will not spend time citing studies showing how exercise improves metabolic markers like cholesterol, glucose, blood pressure, inflammation, endurance, joint mobility, cardiovascular health, and so on. You can easily find information and studies showing a positive correlation between exercise and improvement of each of these conditions. I can't tell you how many patients return to my pharmacy after a recommendation of increased physical activity with their symptoms "magically" improved.

EXERCISE AND DISEASE

Exercise is key to preventing long-term disease. A 2016 study in *JAMA Internal Medicine* that involved 1.4 million people determined that increased physical activity correlates with a lower risk of developing thirteen types of cancer. The main types of cancer affected were esophageal cancer (42% lower risk), liver cancer (27% lower risk), lung cancer (26% lower risk), leukemia (20% lower risk), and breast cancer (10% lower risk). Overall, there was a 7% lower risk of cancers of all types. Diet and smoking status also influenced the results.

Being "physically active" can mean walking, running, or swimming at a regular weekly rate; for example, 150 minutes per week of walking. A study released in April 2016 seems to reveal that women who had cervical cancer had a much lower reported recreational physical activity than those without cervical cancer. (Szender JB et al. Impact of physical inactivity on risk of developing cancer of the uterine cervix: a case control study. *Journal of Lower Genital Tract Disease*)

As I feel it important to give you the best information on this topic, I am delegating a large portion of this chapter to a personal trainer I have had the pleasure of knowing since I came to Baddeck to work as a pharmacist. Her name is Roni Davis.

RONI DAVIS – PERSONAL TRAINER

The role of exercise in preventive medicine is one that's widely misunderstood and incredibly underestimated. But before discussing the benefits, I'd like to dispel a few common misconceptions about the role of exercise in weight loss, as the two are commonly associated.

The huge disconnect, even among health professionals and academics, is the connection between exercise and weight. I am willing to bet that if I stopped a hundred average people on the street and asked them, "Does exercise result in weight loss?" the answer would most likely be yes. This message is driven home by the fitness industry and the media ad nauseam every day.

"Lose Your Love Handles with These Three Simple Exercises"
"5 Minute Belly Fat Workout"
"Trim Those Thighs With This Workout"

We're bombarded with headlines like those everywhere we look, which is part of the problem.

Years ago, I bought a heart rate monitor. It spit out all kinds of numbers like heart rate, obviously, but also the estimated number of calories burned during exercise, based on age, height, and weight. It's important to note that these aren't the most accurate measures in the world. The rate of calorie burn is dependent upon way too many factors for a simple heart rate monitor to determine – but they give a general idea. At any rate, I remember the first time I used the thing. I busted my butt hard. My heart felt like it was being stabbed by my lungs, I was dripping in sweat and hating life pretty bad for a solid fifteen minutes before I looked down at my wrist. Expecting to see a huge number in the "calories burned" area, I was painfully disappointed when I saw the number 70 staring back at me. That's barely even burning off the cream I had in my coffee for breakfast!

I cannot tell you how many times I've had clients work with me for weeks or months with no change in weight. I have a bit of a well-earned reputation for providing tough workouts, so I can promise that during their hour with me two or three times a week, they were suffering and left in a sweaty mess every time. Yet, despite the work, weeks will pass and they see no change in the scale. I hear, "I don't understand. I'm working so much harder than I was. Why isn't the scale moving?" Well, because of my anecdote above about the number of calories that a hard workout actually burns. No matter how many times I explain this fact, people still have trouble accepting it.

A study in 2008 looked at the simple act of walking and its effect on weight loss when diet doesn't change. It looked at several studies and found a remarkable similarity among all of them: walkers lost only an average of one pound for every ten weeks of walking 2000 to 4000 steps per day. (Richardson, CR et al. A Meta-Analysis of Pedometer-Based Walking Interventions and Weight Loss. *Annals of Family Medicine.* 2008 6.1: 69-77. PMC. Web. 23 May 2016)

That's not at all surprising, since walking only burns between 80 and 140 calories an hour for the average person.

Let's look at average calories burned in other forms of exercise. One hour of low-intensity exercise like yoga can burn as little as 200 calories, while an hour of high-intensity, high-impact cardio can burn as much as 1000 calories. However, burning that much is extremely unlikely for someone just starting out, because fitness levels wouldn't allow for pushing oneself hard enough. I'm going to use a mid-range amount of 500 calories as an example in order to do some simple math. Losing one pound of fat requires a calorie burn of 3500. So, you've worked out with a trainer for two hours this week and burned 500 calories at each session for a total extra calorie burn of 1000 calories for the week. That would mean *at best* you'd need three and a half weeks to lose even one pound of fat, if you changed nothing else.

You suffered and sweated, then hurt like heck for days following. Like a lot of people, you didn't look at the meal plan provided to go with your workouts and haven't changed your eating habits because you've worked so hard. You're convinced you're going to see a huge drop in the scale without having to change much. You're exercising now after all, right?

What most people forget is that on Friday you decide to treat yourself with a refreshing iced coffee from your favourite coffee shop. It's only a little cold coffee and you've worked hard this week. Saturday night comes along, and you decide to have a glass of wine to unwind. Sunday brunch has you slipping an extra piece of bacon or two. Now we have to subtract the iced coffee (~500 calories – yep, they can be that much or *more*), glass of wine (~120 calories), and the extra bacon (80–100 calories) from the 1000 you burned during your workout. Those few little extras (which you didn't even really think about!) added about 700 calories back into your week and left you with a caloric deficit of 300 for the week, not the 1000 that you burned at workouts. At this rate, instead of it taking three and a half weeks to lose one pound of fat, it will take over ten weeks to lose just one pound. (Note that I said, "to lose one pound of fat" not "for the scale to drop." I'll explain more on fat loss versus weight loss below.)

As you can see, using exercise alone as a means of weight loss will leave most people sorely disappointed. As a matter of fact, large amounts of weight loss are possible and frequently happen without ever engaging in a minute of exercise – but that doesn't mean exercise isn't a super important part of weight loss attempts – or a healthy lifestyle, for that matter.

Unfortunately, the purpose of exercise has gotten misconstrued over the years.

What is the purpose of exercise? Primarily, to build muscle. Exercise, when done right and combined with proper nutrition, can build muscle, and muscle is your Holy Grail when it comes to weight loss, body composition, belly fat, and even improved health.

Incorporating a proper exercise program, particularly one that includes heavy resistance training, to your weight-loss attempts can mean the difference between weight loss and fat loss. This is a very important distinction.

WEIGHT LOSS AND FAT LOSS

Anyone who's ever started a diet has done so because they wanted to lose fat. There's a *big* difference between "weight loss" and "fat loss." Sadly, everyone is so obsessed with the instant gratification of seeing numbers on a scale drop during weight loss that the majority of mainstream fad diets are designed to cater to this instant gratification instead of teaching us the right way to eliminate fat.

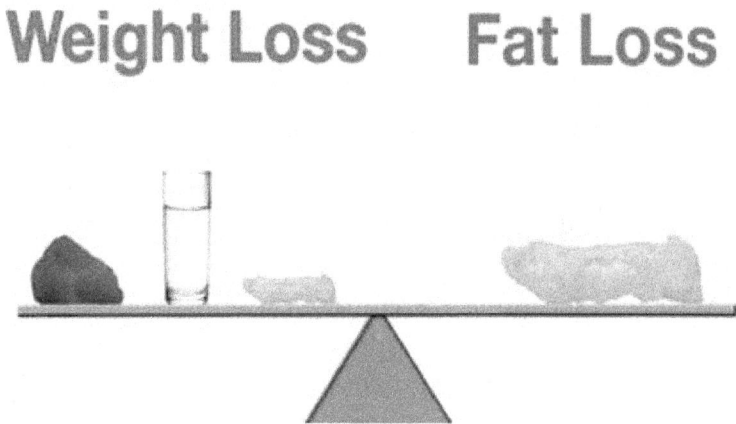

Take a look at the great visual above. If you're going to see the scale go down five pounds, where would you like those five pounds to come from? On the left, you're losing muscle, water, and a little fat. On the right, you're losing all fat.

On the left, weight loss = muscle loss + water loss + fat loss. Under the right conditions the numbers on a scale may drop fairly fast, but that drop is generally accomplished by crash dieting and no (or improper) exercise. As much as 60% of weight loss usually comes from muscle, water, glycogen stores, etc. – everything *but* fat. Weight loss should not be our objective. Weight loss decreases our fitness levels and reduces our strength, our performance, and our energy. It reduces our immunity and makes us look and feel older. And worst of all, weight loss usually destroys our metabolism, making it easier to put weight back on and harder to take it back off the next time.

Now that we understand weight loss, let's look at fat loss.

In stark contrast to weight loss, focusing on fat loss through a proper exercise and nutrition program results in reduction of stored body fat and maintenance or increase of lean tissue (muscle). Fat loss improves fitness levels, increases strength, enhances performance and energy, reduces the risk of disease, keeps our metabolism healthy, and leaves us looking tight, strong, healthy, and youthful.

Weight loss focuses on the scale and sees exercise and even food and calories as the enemy. Fat loss is a focus on everything else with the knowledge that the muscle we maintain or even build during a proper exercise program (combined with proper nutrition) is one of our biggest allies in building healthy, lean bodies that will last.

THE BASICS OF BUILDING MUSCLE

Muscle growth is caused by repeatedly breaking down and rebuilding muscle fibres. Exercise is the catalyst for this process, but only if it's done right.

Damage: First, you must create enough force (resistance/weight) to tear muscle fibres. This can be done by progressively lifting heavier weight, being mindful of and changing rep ranges from time to time, or changing your routine with some frequency so your muscles are continually forced to step up to the new demands. If you don't constantly ask more of them, they have no need to grow. You're also going to need to push them to failure. If you're just mindlessly swinging around a dumbbell and going through the motions of a movement, there's little chance of your workout doing anything for you. Keep the muscle you're working on tight. Focus. Use good form and a weight heavy enough that the last few reps are quite difficult to complete. Remember that you are deliberately trying to create trauma – not just make them burn!

Recovery/Rebuilding: Repairing that trauma requires both fuel and rest. Once you've managed to tear up those muscle fibres, they won't be able to rebuild without the proper amounts of the right nutrients: protein of course, fats, and yes, even carbs! They also require rest, which is why a key element to any successful workout program is providing the correct amount of time before returning to specific muscle groups, and why getting enough sleep should be a priority.

Consistency: Damage and recovery are the building blocks of growth, but actual growth occurs when we stack these blocks on top of one another. We must repeat the damage/progressive overload/recovery cycle over a long period of time. Last, you have to lose some of the fat covering those beautiful muscles, which is where diet and cardio come into play. You can't skip or half-ass any of those things, *especially* if you're starting out with a lot of weight to lose or have lost a lot and feel flabby.

MAIN TYPES OF EXERCISE

It is important to understand that not all exercise is created equal. Different types of exercise are required for different purposes.

The basics are resistance/weight training, cardio, and stretching.

Resistance Training/Weightlifting

Overgrown bodybuilders have given weightlifting a bad rap with the general public over the years. Many people, women in particular, tend to shy away from lifting weights for fear of getting too "bulky." On the contrary, resistance training is key to keeping our bodies healthy, firm, and strong as we age. It's also the key to achieving that much coveted "toned" appearance. I'd be willing to bet almost everyone starting a weight-loss program wants to be "toned," but most people don't even understand the concept. Generally, when people refer to being "toned," they are imagining a firm body with some muscular definition. Women in particular are targeted daily with promises of specially designed yoga or Pilates or other exercise programs that will "tone" their bodies and create "long and lean muscles without bulk." The truth is, weight training is what is really used to achieve this look.

The reality is that the body is made up of different kinds of tissues. When it comes to our physical appearance, two types of tissue matter: muscle and fat. Muscle is lean and firm. It can't be "toned" or "untoned," nor can it become either fatter or leaner. Likewise, fat is soft and cushiony. It cannot become "toned"; there is simply more or less of it on different parts of the body. You cannot turn fat into muscle, and you cannot turn muscle into fat. The two types of tissues are separate, like oil and water.

Muscles are fixed at all ends by tendons and bone, so they absolutely *cannot* be made to assume different lengths or shapes. The length and shape of our muscles is largely genetic and cannot be changed by any type of exercise program. Fat is...well, fat. It's soft and it's what covers our muscles. The term "lean muscle" is thrown around everywhere, and it annoys me as it is redundant. Muscle *is* lean. You cannot have a lean muscle or a fatty muscle. If someone has a lot of muscle but it's not visible, it's because body fat is covering it, not because they have built fat or bulky muscles instead of lean muscles. The more fat we have over our muscles, the less firm our bodies appear, especially if we don't have much muscle underneath.

The only ability muscles have is to either: (1) grow larger and/or become stronger *or* (2) shrink smaller and/or become weaker (this happens naturally as we age, by the way).

We've all seen people who drop large amounts of weight but end up looking like a smaller version of themselves – or worse, like they've been deflated because they are so jiggly. The reason for this is that they have not developed any muscle. They may lose weight, but they don't appear "toned" because they don't have enough muscle under the remaining layer of fat. Think about it – if muscle is the tissue that's firm and we lose weight without building muscle underneath, what do you think we'll be left with? That's right...jiggle.

OTHER BENEFITS OF WEIGHT TRAINING

Body Composition

The basics of toning and weight loss versus fat loss that I've already talked about are rooted in body composition. Body composition is used to describe the percentages of fat, bone, water, and muscle in our bodies. The lower your body fat percentage is, the leaner/firmer your body will appear.

Increased Metabolism

Muscle boosts metabolism. Metabolism is the biochemical process that converts the calories in food and beverages we consume into energy that our bodies use to function. Even at rest, our body needs this energy for all its "hidden" functions, such as breathing (kind of important), circulating blood, adjusting hormone levels, and growing and repairing muscles and cells.

BMR

The number of calories your body uses to carry out just these basic functions of life is known as your Basal Metabolic Rate or BMR. BMR is unique to each individual. Let's examine some of the factors that can affect your BMR:

1. **Size and Body Composition**. The bodies of people who are larger burn more calories. And the bodies of people with more muscle burn more calories, even at rest. This is why muscle is so important to losing belly fat in particular, and why women may notice that the men in their lives have an easier time losing weight. Muscle is what is referred to as "metabolically active" tissue. Even when we are sleeping, muscle is like a furnace burning away fat and calories for us.
2. **Gender**. As just mentioned, men usually have less body fat and more muscle than do women of the same age and weight, thus they tend to burn more calories.
3. **Age**. As we get older, the amount of muscle we have will decrease if we don't work to preserve it. This makes relative body-fat percentages go up – fat accounts for more of your weight, slowing down calorie burning.
4. **Diet**. Hopefully, you have not spent years on yo-yo diets. The term "starvation mode" gets thrown around a lot, but what it refers to is the body's response to prolonged periods of severe calorie restriction. Calorie restriction decreases the body's metabolic rate. This is the worst thing ever for weight loss goals.

We know that our BMR is the amount of energy (calories) we need just to stay alive. We know that it's different for everyone and that it can change. For example, as just mentioned, if you build muscle, your BMR can go up. If that's not the single best reason to weight train for weight loss, I don't know what is. However, similarly, if you lose muscle (diet hard without strength training) your BMR will go down.

How do we know what our BMR is? Short of visiting a lab and taking some very specific tests, it's impossible. There are several formulas that can help us estimate, and there are even BMR calculators available online, but they are largely inaccurate.

At any rate, let's use a basic online BMR calculator and make up an imaginary person to help us illustrate why it's so important to make sure you protect your metabolism.

Let's invent a thirty-year-old female who is five feet six inches tall and weighs 175 pounds. A BMR calculator says her BMR is 1585. This means that just to keep her body alive, without even moving, she needs 1585 calories a day. A bigger, younger woman would need even more.

What happens when her caloric intake drops below her BMR? Say she only eats 1000 calories? Obviously she doesn't die, right? No, her body has to pull those extra calories it needs to avoid death from somewhere. "Oh good, it'll burn off all her fat!" you think. Wrong. Fat stores are our bodies' safety net in times of extreme stress. Our bodies hang on to fat for dear life, and if we are not doing things right, our bodies will burn everything else first and fat last – that "everything else" being muscle. When you drop your calories below your BMR and lose weight, particularly if you're not strength training, you are almost certainly losing mostly muscle with only maybe a little fat.

Now, let's say our hypothetical woman repeats her severe calorie restriction for a long period of time. Her body is hardwired for survival. In the case of severe calorie restriction, a body will adapt by slowing down the metabolism in order to survive on less. So if when she started, her BMR was 1585 and she spends too much time living on 1000, her body will adjust her BMR to 1000. So now, instead of being able to lose weight on 1700 or 1800 calories a day, she needs to be closer to 1000. If she goes below that for too long, it takes even less. This means it will take far fewer calories for the woman to gain weight than it did before. This is a messed-up metabolism – or starvation mode. A person in starvation mode can still lose, but they have to keep dropping caloric intake until there's nothing left, and by that time they have no muscle or energy left either.

As you can see, a healthy metabolism is vital to weight management, and it's absolutely within our control!

Strength
Increased muscle *strength*, power, endurance, and size. One of the best benefits of strength training is right there in the name: strength! Weights help make us stronger for everything. Carrying groceries, piggy-backing the kids around, climbing stairs – literally all everyday tasks are easier when you're stronger.

Flexibility
By working muscles dynamically through a full range of motion, weight training can improve overall *flexibility* and mobility, making simple acts of daily life much easier. Increased flexibility also reduces the risk of back pain, muscle pulls, and other injuries.

Likelihood of Injury
Strength training doesn't just strengthen muscles. It also strengthens tendons, ligaments, and bones. Strong tendons, ligaments, and bones are less likely to give way under stress, thus making them less likely to be injured. Increased bone density and strength also reduces back and knee pain significantly.

Additional Health Benefits of Strength Training

- Increases HDL – High Density Lipoprotein (good cholesterol), and decreases LDL – Low Density Lipoprotein (bad cholesterol).

- Reduces risk of diabetes and insulin needs.
- Lowers risk of cardiovascular disease.
- Lowers high blood pressure.
- Lowers risk of breast cancer – reduces high estrogen levels linked to the disease.
- Decreases or minimizes risk of osteoporosis by building bone mass.
- Reduces symptoms of PMS (Premenstrual Syndrome).
- Reduces stress and anxiety.
- Decreases colds and illness.
- Improves sleep.

CARDIOVASCULAR EXERCISE

Cardio, short for cardiovascular exercise, is basically anything that gets your heart rate up and increases blood circulation. Because cardio forces your heart to work harder, over time it makes your heart stronger. Think of it as strength training for the main engine of your whole body.

Most people think of cardio as a means to burn off excess calories. Since it makes the heart pump faster and the body work harder, cardio will increase the need for energy. Generally speaking, short bursts of high intensity intervals (HIIT) like sprints, for example, will have a far greater caloric burn and impact on metabolism than activities which are steady state, like running at a constant speed. Cardio alone, especially steady-state cardio, is not the best choice for fat loss.

It will likely come as quite a surprise to many people that in terms of fat loss, steady-state activities can actually be counterproductive and can even make your body hold on to its body fat stores.

Running is a phenomenal cardiovascular activity that can play an important role in a weight-loss program – under the right circumstances. When you begin a running program, you will burn an incredible number of calories and it will help dramatically with weight loss because it's not something your body is good at yet. Our bodies are incredibly adaptive machines and quickly become very efficient at doing things we ask them to do on a regular basis. So, if you are going out day after day and doing the same hour of running, along the same route at the same pace, your body learns how to adjust and eventually becomes more efficient – at saving caloric energy, not burning it. This is true of any steady-state cardiovascular exercise.

No matter how evolved we become, our body's primary goal will always be survival. One of the most important survival mechanisms that mammals like us have developed is the conservation of as much fat as possible.

Repeated endurance activities, like running for long durations, put the body into a state that not only forces metabolism to slow, but also decreases energy expenditures from body fat stores. What does that mean? The metabolism slowing down means that you are not burning as many calories. When the energy being used reverts away from fat stores, it means the calories you are burning are coming from sources other than that stubborn fat you are trying so hard to get rid of – sources like our ever-so-precious muscle!

I always recommend cardio, but I hope it is clear that many of the best reasons to engage in cardiovascular activities have nothing to do with weight.

Other Benefits of Cardio

Improved Heart Health
As I touched on already, your heart is a muscle just like any other, and cardio is like strength training for your heart. It will weaken over time if you ignore it, and a weak heart can cause a variety of negative health effects.

Improved Hormonal Profile

Performing cardiovascular exercise also changes the hormonal profile in your body considerably. It releases "feel good" hormones that will help ease symptoms of depression and fatigue. They don't call it "runner's high" for nothing.

Management of Diabetes

Cardio helps improve the body's ability to utilize glycogen – those who do engage in cardio regularly tend to have a better control of their blood sugars and don't see as many swings when compared with those who don't.

STRETCHING

There are two types of stretching – dynamic and static. Dynamic stretching is what we use at the beginning of a workout because it mimics the movements used in the sport or activity and helps to warm up and prepare the body by increasing blood flow and muscle temperature. Have you ever gotten up feeling super stiff in the morning, but after moving around for a few minutes, started to feel more mobile? It's like that. It's important to use dynamic stretching pre-workout, not static stretching.

Static stretching is what most people think of when it comes to stretching. It's the typical stretch, hold for a period of time, and release. It is also what most people tend to do pre-workout, if they bother to stretch at all. Statically stretching a cold muscle may pull or injure it. Think again for a second about that morning you woke up feeling stiff and imagine if you immediately tried to drop down into the splits. It's not going to happen, and you'll likely get up with something pulled and sore. Static stretching is great to use post-workout, however, when muscles are already warm and loose.

The benefit of stretching, obviously, is increased flexibility and mobility in muscles and joints. Don't ever take for granted how important stretching is and how nice it feels to have a body that can move easily through all ranges of motion.

BEYOND WEIGHT MANAGEMENT

"Of all the self-fulfilling prophecies in our culture, the assumption that aging means decline and poor health is probably the deadliest." – Marilyn Ferguson

The old saying "move it or lose it" could not be truer of our bodies. It's a shame that exercise has become so synonymous with weight loss. We forget the real reasons we should all be engaging in some form of regular exercise program – to care for our bodies and stay healthy! Our bodies naturally deteriorate as we age, but the rate and extent to which they do is almost entirely dependent upon how well we care for them and whether or not we work to keep them strong and active. It is 100% within our control to add regular exercise to our lives. In addition to keeping us stronger, more mobile, postponing disease and disability, and even looking tighter and younger as we age, regular exercise can dramatically improve or even eliminate many common health problems.

Studies everywhere prove exercise improves not only self-esteem and mood disorders like depression, but also metabolic markers like cholesterol, glucose, blood pressure, inflammation, endurance, joint mobility, cardiovascular health, chronic back (knee, shoulder, hip, etc.) pain, and so on. Even more convincing than studies, I speak from both personal and professional experience when I tell you I have seen the power of exercise not only in myself but in my clients every single day.

SAMPLE WORKOUT IDEAS

Weight training doesn't have to be scary or require a lot of fancy equipment or even a gym. Below are a few great but very basic compound exercises that will give you an awesome full body workout at any level without requiring anything beyond a couple of dumbbells.

BEGINNER	**INTERMEDIATE**
(2–3 sets of 15–20 reps)	*(3–4 sets of 8–20 reps)*
Body weight squat (or squat to chair)	Weighted squats
Walking lunge	Weighted walking lunge
Bent rows	Bent rows or renegade rows
Overhead press	Overhead press or DB thruster
Push-ups (against a wall or from knees)	Push-ups (from knees or feet)
Supermans	Supermans on a stability ball

Beginner: 2–3 sets of 15–20 reps

Perform 2 to 3 sets of 15 repetitions of each exercise in the beginner column with a one-minute rest between each set, and before beginning each new exercise. This can be repeated as often as every second day, as long as you're making sure to rest one full day between workouts. Attempt to increase the weight slightly each week so you are always asking more of your body. After four to six weeks, increase sets to 3 or 4 and begin to lower rep ranges down to 10 or 12 with some frequency in order to increase weight even more. Once a week, for an added cardio burn, you can speed up your reps a little and perform this as a circuit. That is, repeat all exercises at once, resting for 60 to 90 seconds only after completing them all. This can be repeated 3 or 4 times. This will be tougher than the straight sets so you can lower the weight you'd normally use on each exercise.

Intermediate: 3–4 sets of 8–20 reps

As an intermediate, you can begin decreasing rep ranges and increasing weight. Remember that rep range is decreased in order to allow for weight to be increased. If you've been doing 15 squats with 20 pounds, make sure to increase to 25 or 30 pounds if you're dropping reps down to 8 or 10. Building on the beginner exercise choices, begin incorporating some weights into your squats and lunges. Switch bent rows for renegade rows and give dumbbell thrusters a try in place of the overhead presses. Step up your push-up game by trying some from the floor on your knees if you've been doing them on the wall or try a few from your feet if you've been doing them on your knees. Don't worry if you can only manage one or two, work to increase that amount each time.

Those few basic exercises can be combined to create endless workout ideas for any fitness level. As your fitness level improves, you can even begin to throw in things like sprints, rope jumping, mountain climbers, and squat jumps in between sets to keep your heart rate up for an extra challenge and cardio burst. Always remember to warm up with a light set or two of each exercise before beginning.

It can be helpful to keep track of your workouts by recording the weights, reps, and sets you've done for each exercise every time you work out. Each week, challenge yourself to increase weight, sets, or rep ranges in order to keep progressing.

HEALTHY LOGIC

CHAPTER 5

BIOMARKERS

"Somewhere over the rainbow,
Way up tall, There's a land where
they've never heard of cholesterol."

– ALLAN SHERMAN

The medical community needs some common standards in order to gauge whether a person is healthy or not. There is often a lack of connection between symptoms and lab values. Sometimes these values have little correlation with symptoms, like the lack of symptoms that may occur with high cholesterol. Sometimes people expect symptoms to occur, and when they don't, they ignore their medications, like a high blood pressure measurement. One thing has proven itself in medicine: biomarkers are helpful in objectively and predictively measuring our well-being or risk of developing further adverse health problems.

The best way we have found to make a predictive evaluation of health is through biomarkers, a group of measurements that for the most part are very unrelated but collectively point to one main convergence – your life expectancy. The term biomarker is short for biological marker and has been given many definitions. The best definition I have seen is, "any substance, structure, or process that can be measured in the body or its products and influence or predict the incidence of outcome or disease." (Strimbu K, Tavel JA. What are Biomarkers? *Current Opinion in HIV and AIDS.* 2010;5[6]:463-466. DOI:10.1097/COH.0b013e32833ed177)

Sometimes biomarkers are used in clinical trials as objective measures that provide substitutes or "surrogates" for clinically meaningful end points. In order for a biomarker to be used as a surrogate, there must be a previously established correlation between that biomarker and a health outcome. An example would be measuring blood pressure instead of something else like strokes, which may take much longer to measure in a study. Biomarkers rarely promise a clinical outcome like death, heart attack, or cancer incidence, but some biomarkers have been strongly correlated with such end points. For example, increased cholesterol levels don't necessarily lead to a heart attack, as there are people with normal cholesterol who have heart attacks.

However, cardiac enzyme levels almost certainly show heart damage from myocardial infarctions (heart attacks) or myocarditis.

Some biomarkers are well known to everyone, like blood pressure or blood levels of glucose, triglycerides, and cholesterol. Modern medicine gives a huge focus to these readings and makes them a regular part of most yearly checkups. All of these tests have become undisputed best guesses for a snapshot of what is not only inside your body but the overall state of your health and how healthy you will remain as you age.

Let's take an in-depth look at some of the important biomarkers utilized by your healthcare team when trying to assemble a picture of your health.

WAIST-TO-HIP RATIO

A simple Waist-to-Hip ratio (WHR) can be very powerful in predicting your health in coming years. Applying to people of all ages, it seems like something that is so simple that it couldn't possibly correlate to anything, but having an apple-shaped body can mean that you are more susceptible to health problems than a pear-shaped one. The World Health Organization has recognized this correlation and gives a recommendation for a ratio of 0.85 for women and 0.9 for men as the obesity cut-off point. To calculate your WHR, simply breathe out and measure the widest part around your hips (buttocks) and your waist and divide the waist by the hip circumference. The WHR may be more accurate than the popular body mass index (BMI) in determining obesity. Unfortunately, the number of people who would, by definition, be suddenly classified as obese would increase substantially if we switched from BMI to WHR.

BODY MASS INDEX

A body mass index is often criticized as a number and nothing more. Quite often, it is a number that selectively puts people into an obese category and isn't an accurate measure of health of the individual. Body mass index is a weight-to-height ratio, calculated by dividing one's weight in kilograms by the square of one's height in meters and is used as an indicator of obesity and underweight. (https://www.cdc.gov/healthyweight/assessing/bmi/index.html)

Overall, BMI works best for the average-build adult person. It becomes less accurate when measuring body builders or athletes since they have less body fat, and it also becomes less accurate for children and teens since BMI is based on adult heights. It also fails for women who are pregnant or nursing, since their fat reserves may be altered. Finally, those who are over age sixty-five fall outside regular range cutoffs of the BMI.

BMI takes some criticism because it does not consider body composition as much as it should. You could weigh 250 pounds and have 3% body fat or weigh 130 pounds and have 50% body fat, and BMI might suggest that the second person is in better health, even though most other biomarkers would show that they are at more danger of metabolic issues and chronic disease.

It is becoming more acceptable to allow people to live at a BMI, waist measurement, weight, or any other measurement of weight and obesity that allows them to strike a balance between living as long as possible and living an enjoyable life that isn't made miserable by focusing on a number on the scale.

In fact, both the World Health Organization and the Canadian Medical Association are on record stating that BMI is a rough guide only and not a definition of fitness or overall health. Personally, I consider BMI to be quite irrelevant in determining the health of individual patients. It is more useful for macro-observations of population obesity. Having said this, it is still an important piece of the total puzzle, and if your BMI is elevated or changes, you should be questioning why that is and taking it as a sign that you should be checking what your other biomarkers are, so you have a broader view of the puzzle that is your long-term health.

BASAL METABOLIC RATE

Another important biomarker, especially in follow-up with weight-loss patients, is basal metabolic rate. We have already covered this biomarker extensively in Chapter 4, but in case you're chapter-hopping, here is a brief explanation. BMR is the number of calories you burn at rest in a twenty-four-hour period. If you woke up in the morning and didn't open your eyes, eat, go to the bathroom, or get out of bed until the next morning, you would burn the number of calories equal to your basal metabolic rate. We typically see the BMR drop as an individual loses weight and when body mass drops. Using a machine to find an exact measurement of your BMR is not common, but you can easily estimate your BMR online by inputting your height, weight, and age.

BONE DENSITY

Besides muscle strength, another biomarker very closely tied to overall health is bone density. There are a lot of reasons why we experience a normal decrease in bone density over time, from changes in diet, to nutrient-absorption issues, to medications that are bone unfriendly, to lack of exercise. Bone density is also influenced by hormonal change that normally occurs as you get older. As with all age-related declines, bone density is one of the many biomarkers we try to monitor to prevent us from aging in an unhealthy way. This is fair enough, since an elderly patient with a broken hip who becomes immobile is likely to decline much faster than one who is able to move around.

Decreased bone health leads to fractures, and fractures in the elderly correlate with a decreased life expectancy. We see many more fractures in the elderly than in younger adults. There are an estimated 1.5 million fractures every year in the United States in those aged 50 and older. Fractures can potentially lead to a shortened lifespan or at the very least can result in huge medical expenses.

Resistance training involving weight-bearing seems to benefit over aerobic exercise or even pharmaceutical or supplement choices for bone strength, in that it not only improves balance but muscle strength as well. (Layne JE, Nelson ME. The effects of progressive resistance training on bone density: a review. *Med Sci Sports Exerc.* 1999 Jan;31[1]:25-30)

Telling a patient that they need calcium, Vitamin D, and magnesium for their bones is a no-brainer. One ingredient I see with increasing frequency in these supplements is Vitamin K2. In a three-year study involving 244 postmenopausal women, low-dose Vitamin K2 resulted in improved bone mineral density and bone strength. (*Osteoporosis International.* September 2013, Volume 24, Issue 9, pp 2499-2507)

This supplement has the added benefit of driving the calcium in your body to your bones and away from your arteries where it contributes to plaque formation. (Maresz K., Proper Calcium Use: Vitamin K2 as a Promoter of Bone and Cardiovascular Health. *Integrative Medicine: A Clinician's Journal.* 2015; 14[1]: 34-39)

BLOOD PRESSURE

Blood pressure is the force of circulating blood on the walls of the arteries. Typically, blood pressure is a combination of two measurements: your systolic pressure, measured as the heartbeats, and your diastolic pressure, measured between heartbeats. This is how you end up with two numbers, like 170/110.

The Canadian Heart and Stroke Foundation gives the lowest risk of heart complications to individuals at 120/80 and below and the highest risk at 140/90 and above. Tighter control is needed in diabetics and those with existing cardiovascular disease. In a nutshell, higher blood pressure that is not controlled means decreased life expectancy. (Franco OH, Peeters A, Bonneux L, de Laet C. Blood Pressure in Adulthood and Life Expectancy With Cardiovascular Disease in Men and Women: Life Course Analysis. *Hypertension.* 2005;46: 280-286)

If you don't have a blood pressure machine at home (an $80–$120 investment), you can often access one at your pharmacy. With the accuracy of today's machines and the ease of use, you will get your most accurate pressure in your own environment, rather than sitting for an hour at the doctor's office and then staring at his or her white coat while they measure a blood pressure that has likely been increasing since you got there! Measure your blood pressure at various times during the day and write it down for your next visit to the doctor. If it is elevated during that visit, at least you'll have some backup.

Whenever I am approached in my pharmacy on how to best treat blood pressure, I respond, "At your doctor's office." However, some people say their blood pressure is just a little elevated, and their doctor has given them some time to get it down before their next visit. I always feel badly for people in this situation because all of the expectation built up around the follow-up appointment is very likely to increase their blood pressure!

Before you initiate a conversation about pharmaceutical treatment for blood pressure, get out and walk. There are lots of pedometers and activity trackers out there and they have become quite popular. Everyone seems to be trying to get their 10,000 steps per day. Does this really work to lower blood pressure? Well, back in the year 2000, before it was in vogue, a study conducted on 730 people put this theory to the test. It was found that 10,000 steps per day was effective in lowering blood pressure in those with elevated blood pressure, and this was independent of the duration or intensity of the walking.

What else is available to those who need help lowering their blood pressure? Whey protein supplementation has been shown to lower blood pressure. (Pal S1, Ellis V. The chronic effects of whey proteins on blood pressure, vascular function, and inflammatory markers in overweight individuals. *Obesity [Silver Spring]*. 2010 Jul;18[7]:1354-9. DOI: 10.1038/oby.2009.397. Epub 2009 Nov 5)

Bonito fish protein has also been shown to lower blood pressure by a mechanism similar to the prescription ACE inhibitors. (Fujita H, Yoshikawa M. LKPNM: a prodrug-type ACE-inhibitory peptide derived from fish protein. *Immunopharmacology*. 1999 Oct 15;44[1-2]:123-7)

Again, if for some reason you are thinking of taking your potential or current blood pressure assessment and treatment into your own hands without consulting your doctor about your actions, it probably won't go well. Always be open with your healthcare team regarding what you are doing and share your concerns with them. Do *not* discontinue your medication for your blood pressure in the hopes that physical activity or supplement suggestions will effectively substitute doctor-prescribed therapy.

OMEGA 3

Omega-3 Score

A test that is used less frequently but has claims to correlate with overall health is the Omega-3 score. This is the molecule that changes your cell membranes from rigid to fluid, allowing them to be fully communicative with their surroundings – a key component to contributing to the well-being of the overall organism. There is little doubt the biologic effect omega-3 has on our bodies and health, but what is often in question is the supplementation of this fatty acid and the direct results claimed from it. As someone with a family history of heart disease, I did my own blood fatty acid profile just for my own information. A simple finger-prick test gave me an alarming result:

Omega-3 Index (DBS)	Moderate risk SMI	4.1	% by weight	> 8% = lowest risk sudden MI
Whole Blood Omega 3 Score	High risk	5.2	% by weight	> 6.1% = lowest risk sudden death
AA:EPA Ratio	Inflammatory	13.9		Low ratio = less inflammation

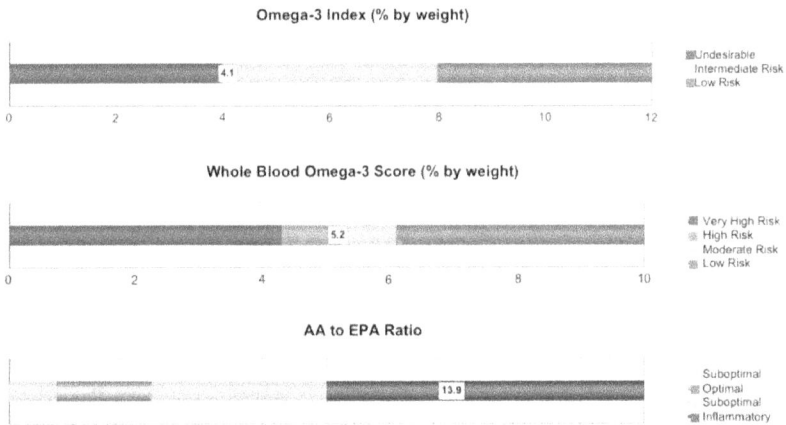

Omega-3 Index (% by weight)

Whole Blood Omega-3 Score (% by weight)

AA to EPA Ratio

As you can see by the results on the bar graph, I was not in good shape. The first graph, the Omega-3 Index, is a measure of EPA and DHA in the red blood cell membrane, expressed as a percent of total RBC weight of fatty acids. A poor score on this index is thought by some to be a strong risk factor of Cardiac Sudden Death Syndrome, and a score above 8% is the treatment goal with EPA and DHA. (von Schacky C, Harris WS. Cardiovascular risk and the Omega-3 Index. *J Cardiovasc Med [Hagerstown]* 2007;8 Suppl 1: S46-9)

The second graph, the Omega-3 Whole Blood Score, is a measure of the major fatty acids in whole blood expressed as a percentage by weight. There is an 80% reduced risk of sudden cardiac death when this number is between 6.15 and 10.2, as compared to a number between 2.1 and 4.3. (Albert CM et al. Blood levels of long-chain n-3 fatty acids and the risk of sudden death. *N*

Engl J Med 2002; 346:1113-1118) As I will describe later, the effect of supplementation is not as clear here. Some studies indicate that omega-3 in your diet has a positive effect on health outcomes such as heart disease; however, more study is necessary. (Siscovick DS et al. Dietary intake and cell membrane levels of long-chain n-3 polyunsaturated fatty acids and the risk of primary cardiac arrest. *JAMA* 1995; 274:1363-1367)

The final graph is the Arachidonic Acid to EPA ratio, an omega-6 to omega-3 ratio. Although the total omega-6 to omega-3 ratio determined in these results was 5:1, the ratio of these two fatty acids was 13:9. Obviously, if omega-6 is inflammatory, clot forming, and pro-cell growth, then you want the ratio to be as low as possible. As this omega-6 to omega-3 ratio increases, there may be an increased risk in disease states such as cardiovascular disease. One interesting disease state that is related to an increase in the omega-6 to omega-3 ratio is depression.

I recently did a talk on cancer prevention for a women's group. Using a map, I demonstrated how and where obesity in the US has increased steadily over the last twenty years. This map shows characteristic trends in the southern states with increased obesity incidence before the rest of the country catches up with them. This map may become the cancer incidence map in twenty years, as obesity is a risk factor for cancer. When I recently looked at the map of depression in the US, it was virtually the same map as the obesity graphic. This is purely observational, and there is no clear correlation between obesity and depression, but it is an interesting similarity to observe and direct further study.

Worldwide, the trend is also similar, with western societies with higher rates of obesity showing a higher incidence of depression, as was the case with cancer incidence. The exception to this trend is India, which has more depression than cancer. We as cave dwellers grew up with an omega-6 to omega-3 ratio of around 1 or slightly higher. The food intake has changed from the paleolithic hunter-gatherer omega-3-rich diet to the Western processed whole-food-deficient diet. Now it's 15:1 to 16.7:1 in western-type diets. (http://www.ncbi.nlm.nih.gov/pubmed/12442909)

This suggests that there is a strong possibility that the way we eat in western-type societies, with omega-6 rich food chains, can lead to many forms of interlinked chronic disease.

Inflammatory conditions like rheumatoid arthritis and asthma improve when the omega-6 to omega-3 ratio is lowered.

This fact leads to an explanation as to how omega-3 can benefit those with pain. Omega-3 acts along the same pathways as anti-inflammatories, just without the bad effects. One must be careful, however, if on blood thinners, as omega-3 can increase bleeding times, for example, for those on warfarin.

In a small study of 250 patients taking fish oil for 75 days on average, 59% discontinued their NSAID medication for pain, and 88% stated that they would continue to take the omega-3 supplement. It was also found that omega-3's effectiveness was equivalent to ibuprofen in pain relief, and no significant side effects were reported. (http://www.ncbi.nlm.nih.gov/pubmed/16531187) I often recommend omega-3 for pain of all types with fairly successful results.

(Artemis P Simopoulos AP. Omega-3 Fatty Acids in Inflammation and Autoimmune Diseases. http://www.ncbi.nlm.nih.gov/pubmed/12480795)

Getting back to the omega-3 blood test I took: After results that indicated an omega-3 deficiency, I began a regimen of daily fish oil supplement that gave me 4 g of combined EPA/DHA for one month. This certainly exceeds the 1 g recommendation most of us see published for the public, but evidence shows that 1 g is not enough to have a real effect on inflammation. Here's why:

After such a whopping dose of omega-3 for a full month, shouldn't I see almost overdose levels of this fatty acid? Apparently not. The three markers are improved, and the omega-6 to omega-3 ratio has improved from 5.1:1 to 3.7:1.

Fatty Acid	Status	Result	Units	Comments
Omega-3 Index (DBS)	Moderate risk SMI	5.4	% by weight	> 8% = lowest risk sudden MI
Whole Blood Omega 3 Score	Moderate risk	5.9	% by weight	> 6.1% = lowest risk sudden death
AA:EPA Ratio	Suboptimal	4.7		Low ratio = less inflammation

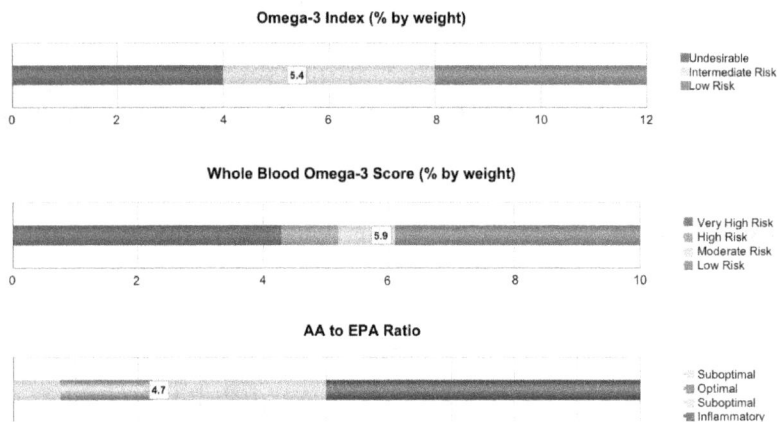

Omega-3 Index (% by weight)

5.4

0   2   4   6   8   10   12

Undesirable
Intermediate Risk
Low Risk

Whole Blood Omega-3 Score (% by weight)

5.9

0   2   4   6   8   10

Very High Risk
High Risk
Moderate Risk
Low Risk

AA to EPA Ratio

4.7

Suboptimal
Optimal
Suboptimal
Inflammatory

A study published in 2018 has shown the value of red-blood-cell-measured omega-3 fatty acid levels in predicting cardiovascular disease. Using the massive Framingham Heart Study Offspring cohort, a study that looked at 2500 participants, it was determined that those with the highest omega scores had a 34% lower risk of death from any cause and a 39% lower risk for incidence of cardiovascular disease. The study also found that the DHA component was more strongly correlated than the EPA component in this reduction. (Harris WS et al. Erythrocyte long-chain omega-2 fatty acid levels are inversely associated with mortality and with incident cardiovascular disease: The Framingham Heart Study. *Journal of Clinical Lipidology* 2018)

While the Framingham Study was a one-point-in-time reading of fatty acid levels, there still appeared to be a clear association. An important caveat to remember is that perhaps those with higher levels of omega-3 in their blood were simply living healthier lifestyles. It was discussed in that paper, however, that the omega-3 levels were a better predictive marker than cholesterol of cardiovascular disease.

What does this all mean about supplementation with fish oil and other sources of omega-3?

A recent meta-analysis that reviewed ten trials and a total of 77,917 subjects determined that there was no effect on fatal or nonfatal coronary heart disease or any major vascular events when supplementing with omega-3. The average period of dosing was about four and a half years. The dose of EPA ranged from 226 mg to 1800 mg per day, and the DHA varied from 0 mg to 1700 mg per day. In this study, over 60% of the test subjects were men at a mean age of 64, two-thirds had a history of CHD, nearly 40% had diabetes, and one-third had a prior stroke. (Aung T et al. Associations of Omega-3 Fatty Acid Supplement Use with Cardiovascular Disease Risks. *JAMA Cardiol.* 2018;3[3]:225-234)

The effects of omega-3 supplementation on otherwise healthy individuals have shown mixed results. The take-home message with omega-3 and prevention of disease now appears to be more complicated than just taking a supplement of fish oil.

As I have stated many times in this book, at my pharmacy I am happy to stock supplements like omega-3 because they may have a positive effect, and there is very little chance of them causing harm. This is how the front store of a pharmacy works. As I learn more about the importance of omega-3 to overall health, I am reminded of the discovery of low vitamin D correlating with many disease states. In both cases, giving yourself a supplement doesn't necessarily mean changing or preventing a disease. It also points to the error we sometimes make in not getting the supplements we need from our food, which gives us other beneficial molecules not found in supplements. Eating healthy is a privilege, and unhealthy eating is not necessarily the fault of the individual. The body needs a myriad of compounds in order to function properly. Given our diet today, which can be far from stellar, we are not getting the proper amount of nutrients without supplementing.

So, what effect did increasing the omega-3 level in my blood have on me in particular? Psychologically, I felt I had accomplished something with regards to a health concern that runs in my family; however, given the evidence that compares the use of supplements over dietary sources, I may not have accomplished anything at all. Given the nature of heart attacks, I may never know. The effect of taking omega-3 supplements is more complicated than reading an advertisement.

HBA1C TEST

Another important blood reading is called your HbA1c. An HbA1c test measures the average amount of glucose that has attached to hemoglobin in your blood over a period of three months. It is a good indicator of pre-diabetes as well as a long-term snapshot of how well diabetes therapy efforts are going. While a glucometer works well for an immediate picture of what's happening this second, an average of the glucose levels is more important. A meta-analysis has shown that HbA1c is a reliable indicator of all-cause mortality and cardiovascular mortality in both diabetic and non-diabetic patients. (http://bmjopen.bmj.com/content/7/7/e015949)

Most physicians agree that they would rather see their diabetic patients with high blood glucose than with low blood glucose. Really tight control is a difficult thing to accomplish unless you have the time (and money) to pursue it.

OTHER BIOMARKERS OF CLINICAL IMPORTANCE

Lipoprotein(a) strongly correlates as a risk factor for cardiovascular disease (CVD). This is a particle that transports cholesterol, fat, and protein. The amount of circulating lipoprotein(a) is determined by your genetics. This type of material increases the risk of plaque buildup that narrows the walls of your arteries. It responds poorly to exercise as well as dietary intervention. Normally we will see these levels remain relatively constant throughout life. Tracking lipoprotein also shows partly how a woman's cardiovascular protection through her natural estrogen production years quickly dwindles to match a man's risk after menopause when estrogen drops off. It is now known that the effect of estrogen on the entire cardiovascular system has incredibly far-reaching effects on prevention of disease in many ways.

Coronary Artery Calcium Score. This shows the increased risk of atherosclerosis or hardening of the arteries that supply the heart and is done with a CT scan. (*Int J Cardiol.* 2017 Jun 1; 236: 473-477 and *BMJ.* 2013; 346: f1654)

CRP (C-Reactive Protein). This is a general marker test for inflammation in the body. Inflammation leads to chronic disease and an overall decreased optimal functioning of body systems. As well, it is the oxidization of the cholesterol in your blood that leads to plaque buildup in your arteries. High levels of CRP also correlate with increases in some psychiatric disorders (*Lancet Psychiatry.* 2016 Dec;3[12]:1147-56), sleep apnea (*Medicine [Baltimore].* 2017 May; 96[19]:e: e6850), and cardiovascular disease (Singh, TP et al. Systematic Review and Meta-Analysis of the Association Between C-Reactive Protein and Major Cardiovascular Events in Patients with Peripheral Artery Disease. *European Journal of Vascular and Endovascular Surgery,* Volume 54, Issue 2, 220-33).

CRP is decreased by exercising. (http://dx.doi.org/10.1136/bjsports-2016-095999)

CONCLUSION

The biomarkers in this chapter are by no means an exhaustive list. I should point out, however, that manipulating some biomarkers such as blood pressure, iron, B12, T4, TSH, INR, and bone density can have immediate results on our health. In contrast, other biomarkers, such as liver function tests, CRP, kidney function, cardiac enzymes, ESR, and PSA are more indicative of something happening upstream that we can't affect as easily.

CHAPTER 6

MICRONUTRIENT DEFICIENCIES

Is cancer really a vitamin D deficiency? Or is vitamin D merely a marker for the disease? Is a lack of zinc a risk factor in getting a cold? Is magnesium deficiency as widespread as we are led to believe? Why do we give calcium supplements if diet should cover everything? Is vitamin K2 important when you are building bones and trying to prevent atherosclerosis at the same time? Do a lack of stomach acid and widespread use of acid-suppressing medications lead to a deficiency in anything?

All of these questions point to a huge issue that is largely unheard of by the general public – nutrient depletions as the result of prescription medications. Yes, just by taking a statin for your cholesterol, you could be creating a deficiency for another necessary nutrient. In fact, it's hard to imagine a medication that isn't a nutrient depleter.

Amazingly, even supplements can cause a depletion in other nutrients. Too much zinc supplementation can cause a depletion of copper, which is why we are now seeing these paired together in a single supplement. Although the depletion of these micro-nutrients has been established as fact, the issue of whether or not these depletions are of clinical significance is worth a closer look. The World Health Organization is keenly aware of the problem of primary micronutrient deficiency overall, particularly as it pertains to lower- or middle-income countries – even without prescription drugs being the cause. (http://www.ncbi.nlm.nih.gov/pmc/articles/PMC2572405/pdf/12751414.pdf)

For the most part, taking short-term medications as directed does not produce significant micronutrient depletions, although depletions can happen that quickly.

Our main concern here is chronic-use medications. Two-thirds of the Canadian population over the age of sixty-five are taking five or more medications, and in the US, over 10% of the overall population admits to using five or more prescription drugs in the last thirty days, according to the Centers for Disease Control and Prevention. Incidentally, when a drug is brought to market, it is tested on individuals, but not in combination with many – or any – medications or other medical conditions. Our assumption is that medications will act the same way in an individual taking anywhere from five to ten medications or when other medical conditions exist. This assumption is important, considering the significant number of people who are on lifelong or at least long-term medications.

See below for more information on specific medications and possible resulting micronutrient depletions. Keep in mind, the following information is not meant to discourage you from taking these medications or to imply that in taking them you are damaging your health. It is merely a guideline of which nutrients you may want to focus on.

Although we may have documented proof that some medications lower your levels of certain nutrients, we may not know the clinical significance of this drop. For example, although acetaminophen can lower the level of glutathione in the body (a key supplement in the antiaging world), the proven effect of this is lacking. All the same, it points toward the need for future research in this area.

PPI & OTHER ACID INHIBITORS

A key class of medications that give rise to nutrient depletions are those given for decreasing acid production in the stomach. The most common in this group is a family of medications called PPIs or proton pump inhibitors. The generic names include omeprazole, rabeprazole, lansoprazole, dexlansoprazole, and pantoprazole. An older group of H2-blockers such as ranitidine, cimetidine, and famotidine also cause nutrient depletions.

Think you're off the hook because you rely on simple over-the-counter antacid liquids and chewable tabs? Nope. Regular use of them could also result in a decrease of some key nutrients.

One of the first nutrients to come up low as the result of acid inhibitor use is vitamin B12, particularly with the PPIs and the H2 blockers. A quick review of the symptoms of B12 deficiency (numbness or tingling in the hands or feet, muscle weakness, depression, or memory loss) may help trigger a question on your next visit to the doctor if you are on an acid-lowering medication. Magnesium is also lowered. This can lead to leg cramps, cardiovascular issues, and flare-ups in asthma. (http://www.medscape.com/viewarticle/803376_3)

Sadly, the acid-lowering medications in the PPI and H2 blocker families were intended to be used short term, for example, for six weeks to heal an ulcer, not to be used "as needed." Most people I see take these medications on a much longer term. Aside from stopping the use of acid inhibitors, there is no simple way to compensate for the nutrient loss they cause.

STATINS

Statins lower cholesterol and may stabilize the insides of your blood vessels. They are widely prescribed and have resulted in longer lives for countless people.

Statins can cause a number of nutrient deficiencies, including vitamin E, CoQ10, and potentially, carnitine. The most common reason I see people come off statins is muscle pain. Small studies have shown the benefit of CoQ10 in resolving muscle pain experienced from statins. Coenzyme Q10 has historically been turned to as the safe and effective treatment for the myalgias sometimes caused from statins. This is not conclusive, but two randomized controlled trials do show significant improvement in relieving this pain using CoQ10. (http://www.medscape.com/viewarticle/776243_1) Based on relatively weak evidence and corresponding clinical response, I'm still not sold, but it is relatively safe to try.

Vitamin E has also been shown in small trials to help, although not consistently. (http://care.diabetesjournals.org/content/36/Supplement_2/S325.full) I always give vitamin E as a tocopherol mixture rather than the D-alpha-tocopherol.

If you are really interested in being on the cutting edge of alternative medicine and trying a therapy based on biochemical and physiological processes without the actual trials to reveal the results, L-carnitine has shown some promise. In susceptible individuals, statins can decrease carnitine. These individuals actually show a genetic pathway that the rest of us don't, whereby carnitine levels are very sensitive to statins being administered. As carnitine has been shown to improve muscle pain from other causes, it is worth a try.

Although carnitine may not be covered by your drug plan, it is safe and may be beneficial, so it's worth a try if the doctor insists on you staying on the statin.

Statins may not necessarily cause deficiencies in vitamin D, but it has been demonstrated that serum vitamin D measurements are often lower in patients who are experiencing statin-induced muscle pain.

As I have mentioned before, we are inundated with studies showing that low vitamin D correlates with many health issues. As we have also said before, we need to be careful to not stretch this into saying that supplementing with vitamin D will cure these issues. There are definitely studies out there that seem to show a benefit with using vitamin D for pain relief, but if it were the miracle drug we think it is, we would be using it more. Clearly, more research needs to be done here.

In an area where physicians are really struggling to keep a patient's cholesterol down, these supplements are safe and worth a try if it means staying on the medication.

ANTIBIOTICS AND PROBIOTICS

What happens when you take antibiotics? Well, if the antibiotic is working, it results in a lower number of bacteria in the body. Unfortunately, this can also mean a reduction of friendly bacteria in the GI tract, which can have a huge impact on your overall health.

Some side effects of antibiotics are just extensions of what they do in your body with regard to levels of all bacteria. When the GI tract is depleted of bacteria, new bacteria can take up residence. This can cause many side effects such as diarrhea or even serious intestinal infections, which then require their own treatment.

Taking probiotics is a common way to repopulate the gut with friendly bacteria and yeast. I use this method in the pharmacy all the time. The conservative Cochrane database has shown benefits of probiotics in preventing antibiotic-associated diarrhea, regardless of the type used. They found the number needed to treat (NNT) was seven. This means that you would need to treat seven people taking antibiotics with the probiotics in order to prevent one from getting diarrhea. Seven treated patients with only one benefitting may seem like kind of a high number, but it is actually pretty good in the prescription and OTC drug world.

In treating antibiotic-associated diarrhea, C. difficile infection (CDI), and travellers' diarrhea, the yeast-derived saccharomyces boulardii has shown great promise. (http://www.ncbi.nlm.nih.gov/pmc/articles/PMC2868213/)

This has the benefit of being a non-bacterial probiotic (it is a yeast) and therefore is unaffected by antibiotics and does not show resistance to antibiotics. A key point to remember here is that not all probiotics are equal in their effects. Some strains seem to show more efficacy than others in their anti-diarrheal effects. It turns out we have a lot more to learn before we can harness the huge untapped potential of probiotics.

ZINC

Zinc is a mineral that is involved in several processes. It is proven to reduce the severity and duration of the common cold. (http://www.thennt.com/nnt/zinc-for-common-cold/) In fact, it is my go-to product for when I am under the weather; and I don't take supplements for the most part. Zinc is crucial for the development of testosterone. It is also crucial in many processes that lead to the development of a healthy baby; for example, DNA synthesis is dependent on zinc availability. (http://www.ncbi.nlm.nih.gov/pubmed/8875519); (http://jn.nutrition.org/content/126/4/842.full.pdf)

Since there is no long-term storage ability for zinc in the body, zinc reserves deplete naturally and require constant dietary input. Levels can become depleted easily if dietary input is deficient and especially if a medication is depleting it. What can cause zinc to drop in a regular population? Oral contraceptives, anti-inflammatory medications, inhaled steroids, NSAIDS, ACE inhibitors, virtually all acid-lowering medications (Rx and OTC), statins, thiazide diuretics, and valproic acid can all lower zinc status with continued use, which is how all of these are normally taken. Not only that, but many of my customers take two or more of these medications together.

For all of the reasons above, zinc is one of the supplements I find myself recommending most at the pharmacy. Keep in mind that excess zinc supplementation can lower copper stores, so cycling your zinc supplements or getting a supplement with both zinc and copper can be a good idea.

As a side note, many of the drugs I listed above can also lower your magnesium levels. Common symptoms of magnesium deficiency are fatigue, difficulty sleeping, and aches and pains. Often, we will treat these with another medication when a trial of a selected mineral may have helped. Multi-drug lists might be reduced by looking at the potential reason a drug is causing a side effect, such as a nutrient deficiency of zinc or magnesium.

ORAL CONTRACEPTIVES

Oral contraceptives (OC) are a type of medication normally taken long-term that can result in depleted nutrient levels.

One common nutrient that becomes depleted in this case is folic acid, which is key in preventing a condition in the developing fetus called spina bifida. Spina bifida is the most common permanent-ly-disabling birth defect in the United States. With this condition, a permanent deformity occurs in the spine of the newborn.

Supplementing with folic acid while on the birth control pill helps in the one-to-ten percent of cases where pregnancy occurs while a woman is on the pill or when a woman goes off the pill because she wishes to become pregnant, then gets pregnant within a month or two. Oral contraceptives have also been shown to lower most of your B vitamins, as well as zinc, selenium, and vitamin A, all key to the optimum function of your thyroid.

Melatonin has also been shown to drop off with long-term oral contraceptive use, which can affect your normal sleep cycle. Other symptoms of low melatonin are restless legs, changes in mood due to drops in serotonin (a metabolite of melatonin), flare-ups of menopause symptoms like hot flashes and palpitations, intestinal spasms, and low-thyroid symptoms. Lack of sleep and a drop in thyroid activity can result in weight gain. Also documented are melatonin's effects on the immune system, inflammation, and as an antioxidant. Put simply, most of the nutrient supplements included in "stress vitamins" are the same ones depleted by oral contraceptives.

The other line of vitamins depleted by OCs are the B vitamins, especially vitamins B2, B6, and B12. As a class, this leads not only to less than desirable red blood cell quantity, but also has negative effects on energy and mood. Most certainly, one of the side effects I see from oral contraceptives is altered mood, likely related to the depletion of B vitamins. During times of emotional and physical stress, B vitamins are your friend.

Magnesium is another micronutrient deficiency found in oral contraceptive users. Magnesium has been shown to decrease over a pregnancy and is thought to be a cause of pre-eclampsia later in pregnancy. Magnesium supplementation helps to bring down the pressure associated with this. (http://www.ncbi.nlm.nih.gov/pmc/articles/PMC2868213/) And low magnesium is implicated in pregnancy-related complications. (http://www.ncbi.nlm.nih.gov/pubmed/25787656)

CONCLUSION

In summary, this chapter has given you a very brief overview of nutrient depletions caused by medications, specifically long-term medications. At the very least, it should point out that side effects that are often considered unchangeable, except with other medications, may be managed with correct supplementation. As we gain a better understanding of medication side effects, we might be able to deal with them by addressing the depletions they cause. There are many credible resources online that discuss this topic. As always, I recommend that you turn to your pharmacist to provide you with the information and point you toward further reading sources. Remember, it's hard to find a medication that doesn't change a vitamin or nutrient level in some way; the key is to determine the significance of that change.

HEALTHY LOGIC

CHAPTER 7

THE IMMUNE SYSTEM

Your immune system is your body's system of defense against harmful microbes. Without it, you are in serious trouble. It is just one of those things that works in the background. Usually, we only notice it when we become sick. The immune system is responsible for protecting us from everything from viruses that cause the common cold to more serious diseases such as cancer. Our immune system can also cause us distress if it is overactive or attacking the wrong things in our body; for example, in the cases of allergies, asthma, and chronic conditions like rheumatoid arthritis. Every living thing has an immune system; even the bacteria that is trying to escape our immune defense system has a system of enzymes ready to defend against whatever tries to harm it.

The human immune system is made up of many parts, including white blood cells, bone marrow, the lymphatic system, the spleen, the thymus, and numerous antibodies.

Our bodies are also protected by our immune system's first line of defense – the external physical barriers that block entry into the body. These barriers consist of the skin, the cornea of the eyes, the mucosal membranes of the digestive system, and the biofilms and membranes that line the respiratory, urinary, and reproductive tracts.

If a pathogen is capable of breaching these barriers, it faces the body's internal immune system. Here, scientists tend to like to break the system into two separate parts, the innate and the adaptive immune system.

THE INNATE IMMUNE SYSTEM

The innate immune system is the main system that an offending organism encounters when it tries to invade a living thing. You may notice some of parts of the innate immune system on your blood requisition when you have lab work done. For example, phagocytes (macrophages, neutrophils, monocytes and dendritic cells) have the ability to physically ingest the offending agent and are natural killer cells ready to kill cancer cells.

Phagocytes get their name from a Greek work that means "to devour." Maybe they were the inspiration for the game Pac-Man, since the specialized white blood cells physically ingest the offending agent.

Some white blood cells release substances that are the principle cause of the inflammatory reaction. One of the molecules released by white blood cells is histamine, which causes arteries to expand and, in the process, results in fluid leaking into surrounding tissue. You may have directly dealt with this inflammatory mediator many times by buying an antihistamine over the counter in your pharmacy to reduce the effects of this one molecule on your body.

THE ADAPTIVE IMMUNE SYSTEM

The adaptive (or acquired or specific) immune system utilizes cells called lymphocytes (such as B cells and T cells), which record "memories" of what the body has been exposed to in the past. The initial exposure of these cells to an invader results in a relatively slow process that leads to acquired immunity whereby the cells of the immune system adapt to the specific invader. The next time that invader appears, the response is much quicker because these cells now remember them from before and take out the invader.

INNATE AND ADAPTIVE WORKING TOGETHER

These two types of immunity also use mediators to mobilize each other. These are messengers that communicate a message from one cell to the next. This includes, but is not limited to, cytokines, which are small proteins involved in cell signaling. It is like a morse code signal between cells that lets another cell know what is happening and what is needed next in the response.

These mediators are mentioned often in preventive medicine, particularly in cancer prevention.

Some cytokines are responsible for your fever when a pathogen or invader enters your body. Some cause dilation of blood vessels and subsequent leaking of fluid into surrounding tissue, allowing both white blood cells and red blood cells to move into the tissues and cause tissue redness and swelling. This is the process that we call inflammation.

INFLAMMATION

Incidentally, what is this thing called inflammation? If I asked you what inflammation was, you might think of a sore joint or an infected eye. The inflammatory process involves a cascade of white blood cells and other chemical mediators that alert the body that somewhere needs healing or protection. Inflammation has many possible triggers.

When inflammation comes as a response to a particular threat or event and then recedes, it is called acute inflammation.

Another part of the immune system that deserves mention is the lymphatic system. The easiest way to understand the lymphatic system is as the body's sewage or drainage system. This open-ended tubular system collects fluid that leaks through capillaries and ends up in the tissues of the body. Some of that fluid naturally returns to general circulation, and some of it is picked up by the lymphatic system. When the lymphatic system is working well, your body has a good handle on its inflammation response.

Inflammation is part of the body's healing response; however, especially in situations where the inflammation response is prolonged, the process can also cause harm to the body.

CHRONIC INFLAMMATION

Although inflammation is necessary to heal, chronic inflammation is what we are referring to when we are talking about the damaging effects of inflammation. Chronic inflammation refers to cases where processes that cause inflammation are sustained for an extended period of time. There are many reasons why one may have systemic inflammation. An increase in the ratio of omega-6 to omega-3, reaction to a certain food, exposure to allergens, heavy metal exposure, infection, and chemical sensitivity are some of the triggers for inflammation. An example of a cause of chronic inflammation is excess fat tissue, which leaves the immune system in a heightened state all the time. Ironically, this reaction leads to more fat storage. We don't know for certain why excess fat tissue triggers an inflammation response, but the occurrence has been well documented.

This reaction can help us understand the relationship between obesity and chronic diseases like arthritis, asthma, diabetes, and heart disease. Each of these diseases is tied very closely to the body's inflammation response. In fact, the whole issue with cholesterol and heart disease is now moving away from the level of HDL, LDL, and triglycerides and more toward a cholesterol particle size and chronic inflammation issue that allows the original plaque to form in place and rupture, resulting in a heart attack.

In a recent study of a large number of centenarians and their offspring, it was determined that inflammation was a key driver to lower life expectancy, and lack of inflammation was common in those that lived to the oldest ages. Your physician may do some simple blood tests, such as SED rate and C-reactive protein (CRP), to measure inflammation.

To understand how inflammation can result in disease, let's take a close look at the formation of a disease called atherosclerosis.

ATHEROSCLEROSIS

Atherosclerosis is a process wherein what we call "plaque" (cholesterol and other fats) begins to build up on the arterial wall. This process starts when part of an artery becomes damaged, triggering an inflammation response in the thin layer inside the blood vessels. Components of the immune system, including pro-inflammatory cytokines and leukocytes, combine with blood lipids and other forms of cholesterol to start a process of plaque buildup. Plaque buildups are dangerous because they restrict your blood flow and can rupture, causing blockages in your arteries and veins, which can result in heart attacks, strokes, and other issues.

How does all of this relate back to inflammation? Well, when you eat what is known as the atherogenic diet (a diet high in cholesterol), you become significantly more likely to develop patches of plaque inside your arteries, which present molecules on their membranes that bind directly to leukocytes, something that doesn't happen with non-inflamed cells.

As I have said before, of the over eighty different autoimmune disorders we see today – multiple sclerosis, lupus, various types of arthritis, Crohn's, pernicious anemia, psoriasis, diabetes, Graves' disease, Hashimoto's, Addison's, fibromyalgia, Meniere's disease, and so on – all might be tracked to a trigger that caused the immune system to react in a way that resulted in one's own tissue being recognized as foreign to one's own immune system. Some would argue that we should only blame our DNA, as most of these conditions are hereditary. Expression of autoimmune disease is complicated. It is likely a combination of many factors, with inflammation affecting the likelihood of expression in a particular genetic disease.

THE IMMUNE SYSTEM AND RHEUMATOID ARTHRITIS

The current model of how rheumatoid arthritis (RA) develops involves most of the mediators and immune cells already discussed in this chapter. This short description should be easier with the established knowledge of previously mentioned players in the immune system.

Rheumatoid arthritis is a condition where the immune system begins to attack tissue surrounding the body's joints. As always, something happens in the body because of a trigger. In this case, an unknown agent (such as mould, bacteria, or a virus) or some type of stimulus (like heavy metal or pesticide) will bind to the receptors on the surface membrane of the phagocytes we call dendritic cells, and the innate immune system will be activated. Dendritic cells then move to the lymph nodes. At this point, the adaptive immune system is activated as the leukocytes (called T cells) notice this presentation of the dendritic cells in the innate system, and a memory is developed for the response.

These T cells produce the interferon and other cytokines, which, you may remember, stimulate inflammation. One of these cytokines is the Tumour Necrosis Factor or TNF we spoke of. TNF binds to receptors on immune cells and inflammatory cells, which are then recruited to your joints.

Here, the immune system looks at your joint like it looks at a pathogen and it attacks it in the hopes of eradicating it. You are then diagnosed with rheumatoid arthritis. We are now treating this disease with medications like etanercept, infliximab, and adalimumab, which bind to the TNF and essentially inactivate it – keeping it away from binding with the immune cells and stopping the pathway from developing further. Damage done to the joints in this self-attack by the immune system becomes irreversible, and as anyone afflicted by RA knows, it can be quite painful and debilitating. A supplement known as natural eggshell membrane is thought to act on the TNF and interleukin aspect of the immune system to help with arthritis. In fact, it has been tested in both rheumatoid and osteoarthritis with favourable results.

Now, a few minutes ago that may have gone clear over your head, but now that you are familiar with a few terms, the process starts to make sense. Another way to understand this process is with an analogy. Let's say John at school starts a nasty rumour to Peter about a classmate we will call George. The rumour is that George has been cheating on his tests. In this case, John starting the cheating rumour is the trigger, and Peter is the innate immune system (dendritic cell) that has the knowledge of the cheating but is not that effective in doing much about the alleged problem, other than elevating the problem to someone more powerful, like a teacher. In truth, George has not been cheating at all, and actually contributes quite valuably to the overall morale of the class. Peter decides to tell the teacher about the problem in the hopes that the teacher has more ability to watch George during testing and will nip anything in the bud if it happens.

The teacher is the adaptive immune system in this case. The adaptive immune system has been alerted to a problem that does not exist. During the next test, the teacher makes a point of watching George for any cheating. The teacher is already biased and predisposed to what might be happening with George. At one point, George happens to look out the window and the teacher mistakenly interprets this action as George trying to look at another student's paper. The teacher then scolds George and removes him from the class and expels him from school. Over the next weeks, the morale of the class goes down because one of their friends who used to keep the class in good cheer is now unfortunately gone. In this case, the class is the knee joint with arthritis and George is the tissue of the joint. With the tissue damaged or removed, the joint doesn't function properly.

This scenario plays out with other interactions with the immune system and other tissues in the body. People with RA are unfortunately twice as likely to have heart disease as those without RA, because the inflammation can also result in blood vessel damage, plaque buildup from cholesterol inside the blood vessels, and inflammation of the heart wall. A heart attack might be harder to notice, since shortness of breath might be attributed to lack of exercise. Similarly, ankle swelling that indicates congestive heart failure might be confused with the inflammation of arthritis. This shows the far-reaching effects of an incorrectly operating immune system.

CHRONIC HEART FAILURE

Chronic heart failure may have its origins in the immune system. The same mediators we have already mentioned may have a direct effect on the tissues of the blood vessels and the heart. You will recall the definitive role that cytokines play in triggering inflammation and other immune responses. In fact, some medications used for heart disease (amlodipine, pentoxifylline, and beta blockers) have been found to help reduce the levels of cytokines, while others (amiodarone, ACE inhibitors, and angiotensin II receptor blockers) help reduce the gene expression of cytokines. (Paulus WJ. Cytokines and heart failure. *Heart Fail Monit.* 2000; 1[2]: 50-6)

The above are medications commonly taken for cardiovascular disease. Another one, atorvastatin, is a statin drug taken to lower cholesterol. Interestingly, it has been found to increase an interleukin that is anti-inflammatory called IL-10, along with increasing the ratio of anti-inflammatory to inflammatory cytokines. It is believed that this has a positive effect in heart function. (Stumpf C et al. Atorvastatin enhances interleukin-10 levels and improves cardiac function in rats after acute myocardial infarction. *Clin Sci (Lond).* 2009 Jan; 116[1]: 45-52. DOI: 10.1042/CS20080042)

THE IMMUNE SYSTEM AND ASTHMA

Asthma is another common and chronic condition that afflicts millions and has treatments that utilize the immune system. Many scientists speculate that asthma and allergies go hand in hand. The genetic and environmental contributions to these conditions form a complex relationship. Now that we have a bit of education on the innate immune system, it makes more sense if we say that there are common genes that are responsible for cytokines, which promote the activation of T cells, which are involved in triggering both asthma and allergic diseases like hay fever and eczema.

Those with asthma know the fear this disease instills. One estimate states that asthma is responsible for one out of 250 deaths worldwide. (Ober C, Tsung-Chieh Y. The Genetics of Asthma and Allergic Disease: A 21st Century Perspective. *Immunological Reviews* 242.1 2011: 10-30. PMC. Web. 5 July 2016)

While it is easy to jump to conclusions that asthma and allergy are the same disease with different presentations (as 80% of children with asthma are also allergic kids), it has also been found that although some genes are responsible for asthma as an allergy pathway, other genes may be responsible for asthma without an allergy component at all.

This is why some asthmatics respond well to medications like montelukast, which deal with the immune system arm of asthma. Montelukast is a drug that blocks the effects of leukotrienes produced by the leukocytes in your immune system, which not only cause the smooth muscles in your lungs to contract but are also associated with mediators like histamines, which increase inflammation.

On the other hand, some asthmatic individuals are unaffected by treatment along allergenic pathways. We may need to treat these people with drugs like salbutamol, which counter the more direct constrictive effect on the muscles of the bronchioles in the lungs without the immune system being treated at all.

Quercetin is a natural compound that shows potential benefits in asthma. Quercetin has been shown to be effective in the treatment of both allergic diseases and asthma. It can reduce the hyperreactivity of the tissue in the lungs and result in bronchodilation. (Joskova M, Franova S, Sadlonova V. Acute bronchodilator effect of quercetin in experimental allergic asthma. *Bratisl Lek Listy.* 2011; 112[1]: 9-12.) Quercetin has been found to use the same mechanism as theophylline and increases relaxation of the same smooth muscles that salbutamol works on to relieve symptoms of asthma. (Townsend EA et al. Quercetin acutely relaxes airway smooth muscle and poten-tiates Beta agonist induced relaxation via dual phosphodiesterase inhibition of plcb and pde4. *Am J Physiol Lung Cell Mol Physiol.* 2013 Sep;305(5): L396-403. DOI: 10.1152/ajplung.00125.2013. Epub 2013 Jul 19)

I specifically mention quercetin here because, as a pharmacist, I can assure you that one of the lingering problems in long-term disease management is the widespread overuse of salbutamol and the family of drugs it belongs to (beta2 agonists). In fact, overuse of these medications leads to the drug losing its effectiveness in dilating the airways in the lungs as the growing inflammation of the tissues eventually constricts the airways to a point that the patient cannot breathe at all. Something that takes the burden off this treatment is a welcome choice in disease management.

SUPPLEMENTS AND THE IMMUNE SYSTEM

We know that immune function can be lowered by many contributing factors, such as certain medications, smoking, alcohol, lack of sleep, lack of exercise, and poor nutrition. So it follows that improving sleep or increasing exercise will help improve or "boost" your immune system.

In the end, it appears you *can* have some effect on your own immune system.

Probiotics
Probiotics have shown to increase your antibody response to the flu shot. (Boge T1, Rémigy M, Vaudaine S, Tanguy J, Bourdet-Sicard R, van der Werf S. A probiotic fermented dairy drink improves antibody response to influenza vaccination in the elderly in two randomised controlled trials. *Vaccine.* 2009 Sep 18;2[41]:5677-84. DOI: 10.1016/j. vaccine.2009.06.094. Epub 2009 Jul 16)

Probiotics are also listed in the favoured group in this database as effective for antibiotic-associated diarrhea, as mentioned earlier. (Hempel S, Newberry SJ, Maher AR, et al. Probiotics for the Prevention and Treatment of Antibiotic-Associated Diarrhea: A

Systematic Review and Meta-analysis. *JAMA*. 2012; 307(18): 1959-1969. DOI:10.1001/jama.2012.3507)

Zinc

The general population doesn't look at the immune system as a cancer preventor; they want to know if it will get rid of their common cold. What does current research tell us about supplement use for this purpose? Overall, the Cochrane database endorses zinc for reducing severity and duration of the common cold. Zinc prevents replication of the rhinovirus and should be started within 24 hours of the first sign of the cold. This is my go-to supplement. It is not to be taken preventatively for the cold, as chronic zinc supplementation can reduce copper levels. (http://onlinelibrary.wiley.com/doi/10.1002/14651858.CD001364.pub4/full)

Echinacea

One supplement that falls short but nonetheless remains popular with my customers is echinacea. The issue with echinacea is the problem of standardizing what exactly is in the bottle you are buying. This results in data that is like paint spatter on a dart board, with some appearing to give benefit and others having no benefit. Preventive use might benefit during the cold and flu season, but again, this is variable and difficult to pin down as to its absolute effectiveness. (http://www.cochrane.org/CD000530/ARI_echinacea-for-preventing-and-treating-the-common-cold)

Vitamin C

Data on Vitamin C is very slightly on the benefit side of the fence when it comes to the common cold. Chronic supplementation seems to help, and it might be beneficial to try on an individual basis. I believe the issue with this supplement is that the dose needed to work is often so high it will cause unfavourable GI side effects. At least it is cheap and relatively harmless, so it checks off the few boxes I use when

recommending supplements. (http://www.cochrane.org/CD000980/
ARI_vitamin-c-for-preventing-and-treating-the-common-cold)

Garlic

Although garlic is widely used as an antibacterial, antiviral, and
antifungal agent, the results experimentally are just not there to
jump on a soapbox and preach about it. The success of garlic may be
due to the promotion of its ability to kill off some things effectively
in a petri dish in the lab, but good quality studies are lacking. This
is not to say that garlic has no effect. In fact, chronic users may
experience a lower number of colds; however, when taken at the
cold's onset, it may have little effect. (http://onlinelibrary.wiley.
com/doi/10.1002/14651858.CD006206.pub3/abstract.)

CONCLUSION

So, as we have seen and will continue to see, there isn't a clear "yes"
or "no" division with respect to the usefulness of supplements in
the immune system. There will always be a separation between
scientific proof and clinical proof. The unstandardized nature of
some supplements muddies the waters regarding the effectiveness
of these products, but when your pharmacist tells you that "in their
experience," this supplement seems to work best for the patients
he or she gives it to, you are normally in a good place. Just make
sure he or she has screened that supplement for interactions with
your meds and medical conditions. A pharmacist who does this is
the type of pharmacist you should gravitate to.

Whether it be animal studies, in vitro studies, human trials, small
studies, or large studies, all of the evidence must be pooled together
to give an informed and safe result. In fact, some interactions we as
pharmacists warn you or your doctor about when we fill your prescription
are based on theoretical but sound science that has never been proven
clinically. Sometimes we need to go with what we know.

HEALTHY LOGIC

CHAPTER 8

CANCER

"Your present circumstances don't determine where you can go; they merely determine where you start."

– NIDO QUBEIN

Cancer doesn't happen overnight. What most people don't understand is that almost everyone has cancerous cells in their body. This is why it was important to preface this chapter with a chapter on the immune system. Your immune system is working every day to remove cancer cells.

What is a cancer cell? A cancer cell is a normal cell that, as the result of a genetic mutation, begins to reproduce uncontrollably. Normal cells in the human body, or in any other multicellular organism, exist to carry out specific functions. At a certain point in its life cycle, a cell will create a copy of its DNA and divide to create a new cell. Genetic mutation usually occurs as the cell is creating this second set of DNA, when a small portion of the cell's genetic code is copied incorrectly.

You are probably quite familiar with the idea of genetic mutation, since it is the backbone of the theory of evolution, but genetic mutation can also result in the creation of cancer cells. Sometimes a mutation occurs in a normal cell so that, instead of performing its proper function, it begins to replicate very quickly or uncontrollably. This is the primary characteristic of cancer. There are thousands of different types of cancer cells, depending on the tissues where they were formed or other characteristics.

Over time, a mass of cancer cells will grow to the point where, in order to survive, it must develop its own blood supply. This is a process called angiogenesis. At this point, the mass of cancer cells generally becomes noticeable as a tumour, and we may begin to say the person "has cancer." There are exceptions to this rule of course; for example, leukemia, wherein cancer cells build up throughout the bloodstream.

If cancer spreads from the tissue where it originally developed to other areas, we say that it has metastasized. It is this type of cancer that we have the hardest time treating, regardless of medication used. Most of our success is in dealing with the initial cancer.

In this chapter, we are going to talk about nutrition and other factors that may influence the immune system's ability to prevent or fight cancer. This is a contentious topic, as some would argue that the genetic mutations that give rise to cancer are almost completely unaffected by changes to external factors like nutrition. Some disagree with this point of view. To understand why, let's look at an analogy:

Let's say that a cell that is about to divide is like a factory. In a factory, workers on an assembly line complete repetitive tasks. The factory always wants to minimize the number of mistakes workers make. We know that to minimize mistakes, workers should be well-rested and properly fed. Their workspace should be clean, well-lit, and properly ventilated. We also want to minimize their exposure to chemicals that could be detrimental to their health. If any of these factors are lacking, we are likely to see mistakes rise.

In the dividing cell, workers are proteins that replicate our genetic code. It stands to reason that without necessary inputs, or if exposed to unwanted toxins or triggers, these proteins may be more likely to make mistakes that result in genetic mutation, and sometimes, that could mean cancer. Before we talk about nutrition, let's develop a snapshot of cancer in the world today.

CANCER IN THE WORLD

The American Cancer Society has determined that one in eight deaths globally is caused by cancer, making it one of the leading causes of death on the planet. A publication by Health Canada in 2013 estimated that one in four people will die of cancer, and two in four will develop the disease. (http://www.cancer.ca/~/media/cancer.ca/cw/publications/canadian%20cancer%20statistics/canadian-cancer-statistics-2013-en.pdf)

When you consider the fact that almost all of us have cancer cells in our body, it becomes quite astounding that three-quarters of us are able to fight off or prevent full-blown cancer by some defense mechanism or mechanisms. In recent years, the overall cancer death rate has declined. Further, cancers that result from infectious agents are dropping. Gastric cancer is one example. The treatment for H. pylori, the bacteria responsible for increased risk of gastric cancer, has been quite effective in decreasing risk. The vaccine against the human papilloma virus (HPV) has also helped to drastically lower rates of cervical cancer and some head and neck cancers.

While survival rates may be increasing, so too are cancer diagnoses. Numbers of cancer patients are increasing yearly. Since 1950, the overall cancer incidence has increased by 44%, and the incidence of some cancers has increased by 100%.

Some might attribute this increase to more comprehensive screening or the fact that human beings are living longer. Of course, the longer we live, the greater chance there is of a glitch happening in our DNA's replication that leads to cancer. So, part of the reason for an increase in at least some cancers can be attributed to the fact that we live longer. However, in contrast to both of these ideas, if we look at cancer rates in children (a population that is not typically screened), their cancer rates are increasing as well.

Dr. David Servan-Schreiber, who has extensively studied the phenomenon of rising cancer rates, has shown that the global distribution of breast cancer is highest in the western and northern geographic regions and those nations that have developed "westernized" lifestyles, such as Israel, South Africa, Australia, New Zealand, and Argentina.

To be clear, rising cancer rates should not be considered a stain on western medicine. There have been great strides made in cancer treatment in the last forty years, including multiple chemotherapies, regimens, earlier detection techniques, better public education on prevention, and better side-effect management. In fact, let's take a moment to examine some of the ways that we treat cancer once we have detected it.

CANCER TREATMENTS

People ask me if they should avoid chemotherapy or radiation and pursue alternative treatments for cancer. Let me be very clear: cancer is not something to be treated with self-care. I support treating cancer with chemotherapy. Unfortunately, chemo does have the side effect of adversely affecting the very immune system that is needed to stave off cancer. If you are highly averse to the idea of using chemicals to kill something in your body, there is a new form of treatment gaining favour in the scientific community called immunotherapy.

In 2018, we saw the first case of a woman with advanced breast cancer that had spread to other parts of her body completely cleared of the disease using immunotherapy. Immunotherapy uses the patient's own immune system to target and kill cancer cells in the body by first taking a biopsy of the tumour. A biopsy simply means removing a small chunk of the tumour tissue. Immune cells that have infiltrated the tumour are extracted, and the tumour tissue is gene-sequenced to determine the main mutations that drive that tumour's growth. Immune cells are then screened for those that best target the tumour's mutations. These immune cells are multiplied artificially, and when they are put back into the patient, they attack and kill the cancer cells and spare healthy cells in the body.

While this sounds like a huge breakthrough, it is important to remember that this type of research has not been around long enough to give us a full enough picture of how to treat every cancer. Not all cancers are the same. Recently, we found completely different results for a rare type of blood cancer called adult T-cell leukemia-lymphoma being treated with an immunotherapy. The drug, called nivolumab (which has been used to treat other cancers), was tried in this type of cancer in twenty patients. This cancer is thought to be caused by a virus, and it is believed that less than 5% of those infected with this virus will go on to develop the cancer. It turned out that three of the patients developed a more aggressive form of the cancer, and the trial was stopped. Obviously, more work needs to be done.

Now that we have an understanding of cancer in the world today, let's begin to discuss some of the factors that may prevent or help fight cancer. All the studies in the world can attempt to predict who will and who won't get cancer, but we all know someone who seemed to live a healthy life and still became afflicted. There is no shortage of claims as to what to take or eat to prevent cancer. Scientific literature abounds with this subject. It's easy to get into a shooting match over what to recommend in both cancer prevention and cancer treatment. One study will say there is no benefit, and the next day the local paper quotes the author of a different study that seems to say the exact opposite.

A Johns Hopkins study recently claimed, "Two-thirds of a wide range of cancer types are largely rooted in bad genetic luck and not simply the results of traits passed down from parents or risk factors like smoking or diet. Random mutations in DNA are largely responsible for the majority of cancers in humans." I am skeptical of this study. If this were entirely true, the chance of getting cancer would be virtually unchanged over time. As we have already discussed, instances of cancer vary considerably across generations as well as across geographic regions.

An example is the apparent role that soy has on the prevention of cancer in the Asian population. More specifically, breast cancer incidence appears to be lower in the Asian population, who appear to consume more soy. In fact, the entire Asian lifestyle makes it virtually impossible to make any conclusion on the effect of soy consumption on breast cancer. There are too many variables involved, including other dietary factors that could affect breast cancer incidence.

Is it possible to make any definitive claims about cancer prevention? Prevention of various types of cancer consistently correlates with consuming more soluble and insoluble fibre and fewer refined carbohydrates, as well as eating more whole foods and fewer processed foods.

Recently, the World Cancer Research Fund and the American Institute for Cancer Research published a third compendium of information about diet and how it relates to the risk of cancer. Their extensive summary demonstrates evidence of various foods and activities leading to increased or decreased risk of various types of cancer. The foods and activities that have shown an effect on cancer risk are as follows:

Colorectal cancer is decreased by eating whole grains, foods with dietary fibre, and dairy products, as well as taking calcium supplements and engaging in moderate physical activity. Alcohol consumption of more than two drinks per day, processed meat, and extra body fat have all been shown to increase this cancer.

Increased intake of fish, fruit, non-starchy vegetables, foods with carotenoids, tea, vitamin D-containing foods, coffee, and foods with isoflavones all seem to result in a limited decrease in various cancers of the GI tract, lung, breast, and bladder.

My favourite target, sugar-sweetened drinks, must be included here as having convincing increased risk of obesity, which is a risk factor for cancer. Sugary drinks join the list of foods that increase cancer risk, along with alcohol and processed meat. Having said this, we need to be mindful of exactly how much processed meat needs to be consumed to actually cause cancer. In a review of more than 800 studies, it was determined that eating 50 grams of processed meat every day increased the risk of colorectal cancer by 18%. This would amount to four bacon strips per day or just one hot dog. In those consuming red meat consistently, colorectal, pancreatic, and prostate cancer are increased from a population average of 5% to a value of 6%, a relatively small amount and not enough to wipe red meat from your diet. (October 26, 2015, *The Lancet Oncology*)

My go-to recommendation is to get your nutrition through a healthy diet. Eating properly not only gives you the vitamins and minerals you need but also the countless other molecules in those foods that aren't found in multivitamins. These extra molecules all work synergistically to help with your health.

What I provide here is a snapshot of current information based on relatively good science. Overall, these are my recommendations: exercise more, avoid processed meat and trans fat, try to stick to a diet heavily leaning toward plants, limit alcohol consumption, and avoid smoking. Unfortunately, not everyone is able to have access to healthy food or exercise daily, and avoiding obesity isn't the easy choice some make it out to be. Each of these recommendations is great, but most people are already familiar with them and are eager to learn specifics.

What about specific supplements in cancer prevention? It's important to be extra careful to not overextend what science tells us.

We have become a society that focuses on the micronutrients of vitamins and minerals, and we forget that there are countless other beneficial molecules in whole foods. For example, there are a thousand potentially beneficial micronutrients in a piece of broccoli or a handful of berries.

This raises an important, if not slightly tangential, point about a question that I receive quite regularly at my pharmacy. Do I consider food to be medicine? No. Medicine is something you take when food isn't doing the job. Do I consider food to be something that when chosen properly might prevent the need for medication, help prevent disease, and help fight disease in conjunction with medication? Sure.

If your definition of medicine as it applies to food means a possible cure or treatment for cancer, then food is not medicine. In fact, it is only something that will prolong suffering as cancer takes over. If your intake of food is carefully chosen to give your body the resources to augment your cancer-fighting regimen with medication, that is great, but food is still not medicine. Now, back to supplements.

You'll recall from chapter one what a cohort study is. Cohort studies follow a group that has been exposed to a variable (such as something in their diet) compared to a group that has not been exposed to that variable. These studies are great for generating discussion on what future studies should look at, but sometimes the biggest miss in a cohort study is that they completely ignore other variables that may influence the outcome. In cohort studies, we merely look back from a distance and see the difference between the two groups compared on one outcome. As we review the supplements in the latter part of this chapter, please remember that most of the information I am citing is coming from cohort studies.

With vitamins, for many it is hard to believe that something like a vitamin can have any effect on cancer, good or bad. There has been no shortage of studies summarized in the media that show the possibility of vitamin supplements (like vitamin E, omega-3 and beta-carotene) causing cancer rather than helping to prevent it. There is a fine line with vitamins on either side of optimal, somewhere between deficiency symptoms and toxicity effects.

The following is a sampling of some information patients may bring to their healthcare professional. As pharmacists, we first need to prevent harm. Second, we try to make recommendations that will generate a best possible outcome, given the evidence. With all patients, we are trying to avoid hype and over-extending the evidence. We need to realize that no one is hiding a cure for anything in order to make money. As well, if any of these products were a home run, we would be using them in treatments. With cancer patients, false hope combined with a few physiological and biochemical principles can result in a family member that quickly turns on you as a snake oil salesperson. Even so, as healthcare professionals, we need to be knowledgeable about any therapy a patient or family member presents to us, regardless of our opinion of it. For this reason, I have compiled the following list:

MULTIVITAMINS

What evidence do we have to show we need multivitamins? The Physicians' Health Study II was a long-term, large-scale, randomized, double-blind, placebo-controlled trial that looked at 14,641 US male physicians over the age of 50. The study measured health outcomes as a factor of adherence to a multivitamin regimen. Adherence to the multivitamin regimen was roughly 75%, so not a daily multivitamin dose for sure. Also, it could be argued that physicians possibly have healthier lifestyles, so the result in the average population could be even more significant. The results showed a statistically significant decrease in cancer in the vitamin group; although, with some specific cancers, the difference was negligible. The vitamins seemed to have a more pronounced effect on cancer recurring in the subjects rather than a first-time diagnosis of cancer.

(Gaziano, JM et al. Multivitamins in the Prevention of Cancer in Men. The Physicians' Health Study II Randomized Controlled Trial. *JAMA*. 2012;308[18]:1871-1880 http://jama.jamanetwork.com/article.aspx?articleid=1380451)

In a randomized, long-term, placebo-controlled trial, investigators found that daily use of multivitamins resulted in a modest but statistically significant reduction of 8% in total cancer incidence. One remarkable anomaly that stood out in this trial was the lack of effect of vitamin usage on prostate cancer. When this type of cancer was removed from the statistical analysis, the total reduction of cancer was 12%. Another finding was that multivitamin use reduced the chance of dying from cancer.

Interestingly, you can probably count on one hand how many conversations with patients in my pharmacy have resulted in my telling them they should take a multivitamin. My main recommendation is to get nutrients from food. Given the problem some have in reaching this goal, they may insist on vitamins. Speak to your pharmacist if you feel you need one.

FOLATE

One study in 2014 looked at the effect folate had on the risk of upper GI cancers. Folate is a supplement that has received a bad reputation lately in its influence on cancer outcomes. It may inhibit or promote carcinogenesis. Small genetic variances in a given population are known as polymorphisms. An example involves genes that function in the folate pathway and have a definite effect on esophageal cancer. A meta-analysis pooled together studies of various types of cancer, using folate and how it measured up to esophageal, gastric, and pancreatic cancers. This systematic review found an association between dietary folate and a decreased risk of esophageal and pancreatic cancers. It did not, however, observe this association between dietary folate and gastric cancer. (Tio M et al. Folate Intake and the Risk of Upper Gastrointestinal Cancers. *J Gastroenterol Hepatol.* 2014; 29[2]: 250-258)

VITAMIN D

Contrary to popular belief, taking vitamin D supplements has not been found to reduce the risk of cancer. There is some evidence of a general lack of understanding about the connection between vitamin D and disease. It's important to remember that vitamin D may merely be a downstream presentation related to the disease process.

Vitamin D is one of the most studied supplements in cancer prevention and treatment. The higher vitamin D levels are upon breast cancer diagnosis, the better the prognosis. Keeping levels at 40 to 60 ng/ml is encouraged for overall health. Women with low levels of this vitamin at diagnosis of breast cancer were 94% more likely to develop metastases and were 73% more likely to die. One theory is that vitamin D deficiency causes cells to become self-adherent, and this prevents stem cells from reproducing rapidly, increasing the chance of a tumour developing. To make matters worse, the chance of metastasis increases as the vitamin D deficiency continues.

This theory also goes on to explain that the measure of how aggressive the disease is can be determined by the level of vitamin D. There are also clinical trials showing better success of vitamin D in cancer outcomes when it is combined with 1500 mg of calcium per day. (Lowry F. Vitamin D Linked to Enhanced Breast Cancer Survival. *Medscape Pharmacists.* March 13, 2014; and Lappe, JM et al. Vitamin D and calcium supplementation reduces cancer risk: results of a randomized trial. *The American Journal of Clinical Nutrition,* Volume 85, Issue 6, 1 June 2007, 1586-91) It is also important to note that low vitamin D levels may just be a downstream effect from something else that led to the disease. If this is true, then supplementing with vitamin D may have no effect in prevention or treatment of the condition.

Similar findings have been found with prostate cancer. There have been claims that vitamin D can stop a tumour in its tracks – a claim that seems far from scientific. These are the kinds of claims we deal with when patients come into the pharmacy. Several observational studies (but not all of them) have demonstrated a lower incidence of total cancers with higher vitamin D status and vitamin D intake and greater sunlight exposure.

There are lots of papers out there that show the disease/low vitamin D connection. Is there a reverse connection where supplementing with the vitamin D could have prevented the diseases? Studies are now showing that not only increased sunlight but also oral supplementation with vitamin D may be useful in preventing many diseases, such as cancer.

(Chustecka Z. Vitamin D Supplements to Protect Against Cancer. *Medscape Pharmacists.* January 17, 2016; and Garland CF et al. The Role of Vitamin D in Cancer Prevention. *Am J Public Health.* 2006 February; 96(2): 252-261)

Vitamin D and Breast Cancer

Another study looked at the effect of vitamin D on breast density when combined with calcium. This was a questionnaire-based study that checked dietary intake. Dietary intake questionnaires are completely at the mercy of whoever is filling them out, but it is interesting to see the results of this type of study. (Berube S et al. Vitamin D, Calcium, and Mammographic Breast Densities. *Cancer Epidemiol Biomarkers Prev.* 2004 Sep;13[9]: 1466-72)

It was determined that the density of the breast tissue decreased with vitamin D and calcium intakes. Breast density is positively correlated with and one of the strongest risk factors for breast cancer, as they are considered nurseries for tumours and difficult to detect using conventional methods. In a separate study, based on questionnaires of food intake, it was interesting to note that although breast cancer incidence was not helped by dietary intake of vitamin D, it was reduced by supplementing with vitamin D. (Anderson LN et al. Vitamin D and calcium intakes and breast cancer risk in pre- and postmenopausal women. *Am J Clin Nutr.* 2010 Jun;91[6]: 1699-707)

We are often told to avoid sun exposure, and that the threat of skin cancer outweighs any benefits of increased vitamin D synthesis and its downstream actions to promote health. In a study that looked at UV-B exposure and cancer rates in the United States, it was determined that the geographic distribution of cancer in that country could be attributed to the exposure to UV radiation, and that vitamin D supplementation and carefully increased sun exposure could prolong life.

(Grant WB. An estimate of premature cancer mortality in the US due to inadequate doses of solar ultraviolet-B radiation. *Cancer.* 2002 Mar 15;94[6]:1867-75)

Vitamin D derivatives have been found to affect the proliferation and differentiation of cancer cells; and in a study based in Norway, it was observed that levels of vitamin D were higher in the summer and fall, and that survival rates of various types of cancer were better when the cancer was diagnosed during these months than in the winter. (Porojnicu AC. Seasonal and geographical variations in lung cancer prognosis in Norway. Does Vitamin D from the sun play a role? *Lung Cancer.* 2007 Mar;55[3]: 263-70.)

Although this is observational, it was also noted that high vitamin D intake in the summer and low vitamin D intake in the winter resulted in significant outcome changes in two separate studies (one in the US and one in the UK).

Although I hesitate to recommend vitamin D as a viable over-the-counter cancer treatment, I can certainly share the evidence that points to its usefulness. We must also be mindful that a higher vitamin D status in a patient may simply be the result of a healthy individual who looks after themself.

Keep in mind that promoting Vitamin D for the prevention of cancer isn't something your healthcare professional can do. In fact, without knowing what your individual vitamin D levels are, it is a moot point to even supplement. Before you buy vitamin D, remember that much less than 10% of the Canadian population is severely deficient in vitamin D.

VITAMIN C

High doses of vitamin C have been demanded and used by some in cancer treatment. Often this is given by IV to obtain the concentrations needed. Fortunately, toxic effects are often not felt when the IV dose is given for what is believed to be an "anticancer effect."

The argument sometimes given to the physician is that the concept of programmed cell death or apoptosis (the body's way of removing cells that are beyond repair) is significantly induced by vitamin C at sufficient concentrations in the blood. (Park S. The Effects of High Concentrations of Vitamin C on Cancer Cells. *Nutrients.* 2013 Sep; 5[9]: 3496-3505)

Most people consider vitamin C important for preventing the cold or flu. Linus Pauling stated, "You can trace every sickness, every disease, and every ailment to a mineral deficiency." It was Mr. Pauling who made popular the concept of megadoses of vitamin C daily. Reportedly, he took 12 grams of the vitamin daily and increased to 40 grams when the cold symptoms occurred. The gastrointestinal effects of such a dose can be unbearable.

Unfortunately for Pauling and for the vitamin C movement, he died, ironically, of prostate cancer. It is not the purpose of this book to determine whether or not vitamin C helps with the common cold. On paper, this vitamin has many important characteristics that lend it to beating cancer. There is however, enough in the literature to fill an entire book on questioning the usefulness of this vitamin in cancer.

One thing is clear: Vitamin C use for cancer warrants further study. (Padayatty SJ. Intravenously administered vitamin C as cancer therapy: three cases. *CMAJ*. March 28, 2006 174 [7] 937-942; and Riordan HD. Intravenous Vitamin C as a Chemotherapy Agent: A Report on Clinical Cases. *P R Health Sci J*. 2004 Jun;23[2]:115-8.)

Definitely, interest in Vitamin C is increasing with traditional therapy caregivers. Practitioners often field questions regarding the use of this vitamin for cancer treatment. In truth, most oncologists will not condone the use of this vitamin for cancer treatment, although some will allow it to appease the patient.

One recent Netherlands Cohort Study looked at the effects of vitamin C in head and neck cancer and found a clear benefit in the prevention of these two cancers and subtypes. Although some studies have shown ambiguity in the benefits of vitamin C with cancer, the studies that show verification of pathways that could lead to success in cancer treatment are certainly interesting. If there was an obvious success with this supplement though, we would be using it already, especially given the chance it has been given in the literature.

OMEGA 3

It's hard to imagine a biologic system that doesn't benefit from omega-3 fatty acids. Most recently, a 2014 study set out to determine whether omega-3 fatty acids exert short-term inhibitory effects on growth factor signalling in human prostate cancer cell lines, and therefore have an inhibitory effect on the growth of the prostate cancer cells. (Liu Z et al. Omega-3 Fatty Acids and other FFA4 Agonists Inhibit Growth Factor Signalling in Human Prostate Cancer Cells. *JPET* #218974 Dec 9, 2014)

Due to the proven nature of omega-3 fatty acids to have an anti-proliferative effect on cell growth, the opposing effects of omega-6 and the increasing ratio of omega-6 to omega-3 in Western-type diets, it is not surprising to try to correlate this increase with the rate of cancer in these societies. Further, the positive effect of omega-3 on the immune system is well known. (Gutierrez S et al. Effects of Omega-3 fatty acids on immune cells. *Int J Mol Sci.* 2019 Oct; 20(20):5028)

An active immune system is what keeps us all from "having cancer," even though we all have active cancer cells in our bodies. Visually, we can see the effects of an active immune system on cancer cells. In a healthy immune system, the cancer cells are devoured by white blood cells, and omega-3 contributes to a healthy immune system. A recent study in the *Journal of Pharmacology and Experimental Therapeutics* on the effects of omega-3 on cancer showed that the growth and spread of prostate cancer cells was inhibited by omega-3. It appears that there is a receptor that omega-3 binds to that results in signalling to inhibit growth factors, which results in suppressed cancer cell proliferation.

Keep in mind that genetics are not entirely to blame for prostate cancer. When, for example, Japanese men, a population with a low incidence of prostate cancer, or Chinese women, a population with a low incidence of breast cancer, move to North America, these populations begin to experience an increase in these cancers.

VITAMIN E

One hotly debated topic is the role vitamin E has on cancer, especially prostate cancer. Pick up a bottle of vitamin E in any store that sells it – grocery, big box, or pharmacy. What does the small print say for the active ingredient of that bottle of "vitamin E"? Well, probably more than 99 times out of 100, that bottle's ingredient is listed as d-alpha-tocopherol. Vitamin E is an interesting complex of many molecules called tocopherols (alpha, beta, delta, and gamma fractions) and tocotrienols (also alpha, beta, delta, and gamma). In particular, the tocotrienols have been shown to provide greater anticancer effects. The gamma and delta tocotrienols of this antioxidant have shown anti-proliferative effects against breast cancer, liver cancer, colon cancer, gastric adenocarcinoma, prostate cancer, and lung cancer, and are actively involved in removing old and damaged cells from the body.

(Lim SW et al. Cytotoxicity and apoptotic activities of alpha-, gamma- and delta-tocotrienol isomers on human cancer cells. *BMC Complement Altern Med.* 2014 Dec 6; 14:469)

However, when we look at all of the studies done to date, it has been difficult to correlate the theoretical effect of vitamin E on cancer in the real world. Although some studies seem to show a benefit, others seem to contradict those studies.

It doesn't take long to find studies that look unfavourably on vitamin E and cancer, particularly prostate cancer. A closer look at these studies reveals the form of this vitamin as the d-alpha tocopherol form. This is the type of study that makes its way to your news and spreads its way around the conversations at work and with the doctor and can even infiltrate recommendations to the medical community at large. The take-home message is to get a vitamin E supplement that has a mix of tocopherols and tocotrienols or focus on getting this nutrient from your food. Wheat germ, sunflower seeds, almonds, beet greens, spinach, and red bell pepper are just a few common examples of foods containing vitamin E.

The alpha-tocopherol isomer of vitamin E is the only one found in human plasma. The alpha-tocopherol molecule has seven stereoisomers on its own to add to the number of possible vitamin E molecules in nature. This is referred to as "natural" or "d-alpha" tocopherol. This is the reason we see this molecule supplemented as vitamin E in the supplement aisle.

Several studies have been done to verify the theoretical effect of vitamin E on cancer at the cell nucleus level. As always, the proof is in the studies that demonstrate that administration of substance A reduces disease B (in this case vitamin E and cancer). As I have mentioned, I just don't think we are there yet in our knowledge based on scientific studies.

The topic "Cancer and Vitamins" contains a minefield of studies with seemingly opposite conclusions. A pooled analysis of ten cohort studies in 2015 concluded that vitamins A, C, E, and folate had no major influence on ovarian cancer risk when consumed in adulthood. (Koushic A. Intake of vitamins A, C, and E and folate and the risk of ovarian cancer in a pooled analysis of 10 cohort studies. *Cancer Causes Control.* 2015 Sep; 26[9]: 1315-27)

As is common with this type of study, dietary questionnaires were used to evaluate dietary vitamin intake. Cancer can be caused by both inadequate nutrition and obesity (two terms not mutually exclusive). (Busch C. Epigenetic activities of flavonoids in the prevention and treatment of cancer. *Clin Epigenetics.* 2015; 7[1]: 64)

Obesity is a very under-recognized risk factor for cancer (Ligibel JA. American Society of Clinical Oncology position statement on obesity and cancer. *J Clin Oncol.* 2014 Nov 1;32[31]: 3568-74). The inflammation supplied by fat cells in the body contributes to an overall increased risk of disease that is independent of the mere fact that the patient carries around extra weight.

One supplement that appears to be harmful in cancer incidence is beta-carotene supplements, particularly with lung cancer. It is important to remember that although vitamins are supplied from outside of the body and that we need them to live, more doesn't necessarily mean better. I recommend you have a discussion with your pharmacist on the risks and benefits associated with various vitamins.

CANCER PREVENTION WITH "NUTRACEUTICALS"

Cancer prevention with natural products is a hot topic. Nutraceutical is a term used to describe any product derived from food that may have specific health benefits. This is an area where a pharmacist must tread lightly. We are never going to claim, "If you take this, you won't get cancer." We can, however, have an educated discussion with the patient about what science currently has to say about cancer prevention and these products, and even go as far as giving personal opinions on what we think, based on research and clinical experience.

Carrying nutraceutical products in a pharmacy does not mean a pharmacist backs up the patient's belief that they are proven to prevent cancer. It does provide an opportunity for discussion, however, of more proven ways that we know of.

Naturally occurring compounds in food have been studied for their effects in preventing cancer from progressing. These compounds have several ways to fight these early steps in cancer's progression. This should not be mistaken as my endorsement of these compounds as primary cancer fighters; after all, we have conventional treatments for this, even though they can be brutally difficult on the patient.

Instead, I would make the point that if you have a cancer diagnosis and are lucky enough to defeat it with conventional therapies, then what is stopping the cancer from returning, unless you change your life in some way to give your body the resources to fight its return?

My feeling on individual nutrients is that nature intends them to be taken with the hundreds or thousands of other nutrients in whole food. However, the amount needed to match the quantity used in a study might be difficult to consume without a supplement. This might lead a person to lean toward a supplement instead of relying totally on food, like we do for calcium, folic acid, iron, and B12 supplementation for other uses.

Here are some of the more popular ingredients patients discuss with me at the pharmacy. When reviewing these, keep in mind this is not an endorsement to take these supplements as a cancer fighter or preventer. Nothing beats a good quality study that proves life expectancy is extended. Although these supplements may lack studies with this end point, the studies to date are intriguing and help explain the appeal of such products. One other thing to be mindful of is the fact that some studies are in vitro (in a test tube or petri dish) and not in vivo – used in a living being. Of course, these results aren't interchangeable.

Indole-3-Carbinol (I3C), DIM, and Sulforaphane

Found in cruciferous vegetables such as broccoli, cabbage, cauliflower, Brussels sprouts, kale, and bok choy, this supplement has been used for quite some time to help metabolize estrogen into favourable (less carcinogenic) metabolites. It also exhibits potent anticancer properties in many types of cancer. In doses greater than 400 microM, it induced apoptosis (programmed cell death) and at lower doses (less than 200 microM), it repressed cancer cell growth. Through this programmed cell death, it was shown to help prevent cancer. In human studies, it had a synergistic effect with chemotherapy. Note it is important to check with your healthcare professionals if you are taking *anything* while treating cancer, and it is *not* okay to substitute something you buy over the counter for your prescribed treatment.

Indole-3-carbinol (I3C) increases apoptosis, represses growth of cancer cells, and enhances adenovirus-mediated oncolysis. (Chen L, Cheng PH, Rao XM, McMasters KM, Zhou HS. *Cancer Biol Ther.* 2014 Sep 1; 15(9): 1256-67. DOI: 10.4161/cbt.29690. Epub 2014 Jun 27)

In a review of 87 case control and seven cohort studies done in the mid-90s, the effect of eating brassica vegetables was investigated and found to have a clear inverse correlation with lung, stomach, colon, and rectal cancers. These vegetables include broccoli, collard greens, brussels sprouts, cabbage, cauliflower, kale, and turnips. The metabolism of the glucosinolates in these vegetables after consumption leads to various compounds with anti-carcinogenic activity. Caution: these compounds are water-soluble and leach out of the vegetable in cooking processes that use boiling water. High heat will reduce them as well, so be sure to not overcook them.

Resveratrol

Found in red grapes, peanuts and peanut butter, dark chocolate, and blueberries, resveratrol is another compound that induces apoptosis and reduces cell proliferation. It can suppress the growth of new blood vessels, which is a key component to tumour growth. It has antioxidant, anti-inflammatory, and antiproliferative properties, which are all beneficial against various types of cancer. (Gagliano N et all. The potential of resveratrol against human gliomas. *Anticancer Drugs*. 2009 Dec, 21[2]: 140-50)

This compound is a topic of discussion with patients often as "that ingredient in red wine," as they refer to this phytoalexin, and yet another reason to drink a glass of wine so as to prevent inflammation. Note you should not initiate drinking wine for any medical reason you have heard on the news. The recommendations are still one drink max per day for women and two for men.

(Bråkenhielm E, Cao R, Cao Y. Suppression of angiogenesis, tumour growth, and wound healing by resveratrol, a natural compound in red wine and grapes. *FASEB J*. 2001 Aug; 15(10): 1798-800)

(Banerjee S1, Bueso-Ramos C, Aggarwal BB. Suppression of 7,12-dimethylbenz(a)anthracene-induced mammary carcinogenesis in rats by resveratrol: role of nuclear factor-kappaB, cyclooxygenase

2, and matrix metalloprotease 9. *Cancer Res.* 2002 Sep 1; 62[17]: 4945-54)

(Zhao W, Bao P, Qi H, You H. Resveratrol down-regulates survivin and induces apoptosis in human multidrug-resistant SPC-A-1/CDDP cells. *Oncol Rep.* 2010 Jan; 23[1]: 279-86)

Astaxanthin

Found in krill, algae, red trout, salmon, crab, lobster, and shrimp, astaxanthin has also been shown in studies to exhibit anti-inflammatory and anticancer effects by inducing apoptosis by modulating the expressions of various cell mediators. Programmed cell death is an important factor in dealing not only with cancer prevention but also cancer treatment because it allows cells to die in a timely manner before they develop bad habits or transmit bad habits to other cells. A theory in cancer development is the concept of the extracellular matrix (ECM), a complicated milieu that continually transmits signals to the cell. This theory states the ECM is much more important than the inside of the cell and nucleus, which merely does what its environment in the ECM tells it to do. The healthier the ECM, the lower the chance of cancer developing. Astaxanthin works along these pathways.

(Nagendraprabhu P, Sudhandiran G. Astaxanthin inhibits tumour invasion by decreasing extracellular matrix production and induces apoptosis in experimental rat colon carcinogenesis by modulating the expressions of ERK-2, NF-B and COX-2. *Invest New Drugs*, 29 (2011), 207-224)

Curcumin

Curcumin is found as a spice on its own or in turmeric. A compound that is already used clinically in cancer prevention and treatment, curcumin has been shown to decrease tumour size in existing cancers as well as reduce tumour incidence in mice that were given colorectal cancer. Remember that just because something happens in rodents doesn't necessarily mean it happens in humans, but it's an interesting finding, nonetheless. Inflammation is closely connected to tumour production. (Menon, VP et al. Antioxidant and anti-inflammatory properties of curcumin. *Adv Exp Med Biol.* 2007; 595:105-25)

Curcumin has a long history as an anecdotal herbal remedy for many diseases, but in cancer prevention, it appears to have a multifactorial antioxidant and anti-inflammatory approach to fighting cancer. Its drawback is its low absorption and subsequent bioavailability when taken orally. Despite this, therapeutic levels have been achieved, and promising results have been shown. In cancers of the digestive system, oral, esophageal, stomach, intestine, pancreas, and liver cancers can all be affected by curcumin as has been shown by animal, human, and petri dish studies. (Rajasekar SA. Therapeutic potential of curcumin in gastrointestinal diseases. *World J Gastrointest Pathophysiol.* 2011 Feb 15; 2[1]: 1-14)

Programmed cell death and other processes needed to quench cancer progression are found in this spice. Various curcumin analogues have been used with even better absorption and more promising results.

(Huang MT, Lou YR, Ma W, Newmark HL, Reuhl KR, Conney AH. Inhibitory effects of dietary curcumin on fore stomach, duodenal and colon carcinogenesis in mice. *Cancer Res.* 54 1994, 5841-47)

(Wang XF, Wang QD, Ives KL, Evers BM. Curcumin inhibits neurotensin-mediated interleukin-8 production and migration of HCT116 human colon cancer cells. *Clin Cancer Res*, 12 2006, 5346–5355)

(Shankar S, Srivastava RK. Involvement of Bcl-2 family members, phosphatidylinositol 3⊠-kinase/AKT and mitochondrial p53 in curcumin (diferuloylmethane)-induced apoptosis in prostate cancer. *Int J Oncol.* 2007 Apr; 30[4]: 905-18)

Probiotics

With or without prebiotic support, probiotics have been shown to stimulate the immune system. Probiotics are one of the OTC supplements I am most often asked about for all disorders. Using probiotics is such a complicated matter when you are trying to mimic studies that its effectiveness is often overblown. Much of our immune health comes directly from our gastrointestinal health. Probiotics have been shown to inhibit tumour growth in several cancers, not just bowel. Obviously, the best result comes from a properly maintained bowel, so all input into the digestive system can affect this immune result. A hostile environment is more likely in the bowel if alcohol intake is not addressed, sources of metal toxicity are not dealt with, sugar consumption (refined carbohydrates) is not kept in check, acid-lowering medications are taken (which allows almost anything to grow in the gut), or insoluble fibre is low in the diet. When it comes to diet, a continual pattern of dietary fibre intake is key, rather than sporadic use of a fibre supplement. All of these dietary measures must be addressed, or probiotic supplementation will be a wasted effort.

LeBlanc A, Matar C, Perdigo G. The Application of Probiotics in Cancer. *British Journal of Nutrition.* 2007, 98[1]: S105–S110

Saikali J, Picard C, Freitas, M, Holt P. Fermented Milks, Probiotic Cultures, and Colon Cancer. *Nutrition and Cancer.* 2004, 49[1]: 14-24

Sanders M. Probiotics. *Food Technology.* 1999. 53[11]: 67-77

Shankar S, Lanza E. Dietary fiber and cancer prevention. *Hematol Oncol Clin North Am.* 1991 Feb; 5[1]: 25-41.

Journal of Oncology. Volume 2012 Article ID 192464, 23 pages

Campbell TC, Campbell TM, The China Study. *Benelli Books.* 2004

Quercetin

Quercetin is **a flavonoid found in onions, fresh tarragon, buckwheat, cocoa powder, raw cranberries, capers, black plums, and**

blueberries. One interesting note on nutraceuticals and supplements in cancer research is that results can conflict quite often because the bioavailability of the given supplement is such that it's difficult to reach therapeutic levels when given individually. However, when combined with other supplements or medications, the effectiveness of each increases due to the interaction with the others. Quercetin is an excellent example of a compound that appears to become more effective in the presence of other supplements. One such studied example is the combination of EGCG, resveratrol and quercetin, which are effective in lower doses when given together to fight cancer. (Aras A. Targeting cancer with nano-bullets: curcumin, EGCG, resveratrol and quercetin on flying carpets. *Asian Pac J Cancer Prev.* 2014; 15[9]: 3865-71) A 2013 study demonstrated the ability of quercetin to increase the chemosensitivity of breast cancer cells to doxorubicin. (Li, SZ. The effect of quercetin on doxorubicin cytotoxicity in human breast cancer cells. *Anticancer Agents Med Chem.* 2013 Feb; 13[2]: 352-5)

This flavonoid is found in many foods and is a very potent antioxidant. In a couple of animal studies, however, quercetin was shown to exacerbate estrogen-induced breast tumours and kidney tumours induced by the same hormone. It also has the possibility of enhancing cancer cell proliferation at low concentrations but is cytotoxic to the same cells at higher concentrations. (Robaszkiewicz A, Balcerczyk A, Bartosz G. Antioxidative and prooxidative effects of quercetin on A549 cells. *Cell Biol Int.*, 2007, 31[10], 1245-1250)

Quercetin has also shown pronounced programmed cell death in some leukemia patients. We must be cautious with antioxidants. Although the body definitely needs them to ward off free radicals that can do damage to our bodies, too much of an antioxidant may not be friendly on the body.

ECGC

A catechin (epigallocatechin-3-gallate), **found in green tea leaves**, this compound has been studied with skin, gastric, and colon cancer with interesting results. Its effects on angiogenesis or new blood vessel growth may be how this compound works to prevent progression of cancer. In pancreatic cancer cells, it has been shown to reduce tumour volume, proliferation, angiogenesis, and induced apoptosis.

(Mamede AC. The Role of Vitamins in Cancer: A Review. *Nutrition and Cancer.* 63:4, 479-494)

Other Helpful Compounds Found in Whole Foods

Other compounds like **lycopene** (from tomatoes), **genistein** (from soy), and **sulforaphane** (from cruciferous vegetables) have all been shown to have an anticancer effect in theory. They all show promise, which accentuates the recommendation to consume real food, not only to get the possible benefit from these molecules but also from the thousands of other ingredients in real food.

So, above is a sampling of compounds found in whole foods that have been demonstrated to not only help prevent cancer but also fight it, and you can just go to your grocery store and shop for foods that contain these compounds. In fact, I actually filmed a healthy grocery shopping tour (free to watch on YouTube) to help guide healthy shopping decisions, and I will go into greater detail on this topic later on in the book.

Which foods should you be buying to get these benefits? Many studies have tried to connect a healthier diet to a reduction in cancer, with respect to the above-mentioned compounds found naturally in whole foods. Not all have shown the same results. I have read multiple cohort studies that were unable to find a correlation between, for example, instance of prostate cancer in middle-aged men and their consumption of healthy fruits and vegetables.

One interesting study suggested that although there was no benefit to eating tomatoes or fruit, there was a benefit in eating yellow, orange, and cruciferous vegetables, especially in advanced cases. (Kolonel LN et al. Vegetables, Fruits, Legumes and Prostate Cancer: A Multiethnic Case-Control Study. *Cancer Epidemiological Biomarkers Prev.* 2000. Aug; 9[8]: 793-804)

Another study that utilized the data from three Canadian case control studies and dietary intake interviews found that eating green vegetables, tomatoes, beans, lentils, nuts, and cruciferous vegetables led to lower incidence of prostate cancer.

If you are looking for a cookie-cutter answer for which foods do what for cancer prevention, it is easy to find one study that provides you with some suggestions, but it is very hard to find multiple studies that back up your first study's conclusion. There are different types of cancers and different types of compounds, in different types of food, working through different mechanisms.

I sometimes feel frustrated when asked to make a recommendation on how eating the correct food affects cancer. There is simply no flip-on, flip-off switch for fighting cancer. In truth, we just aren't at enough of a level of understanding to firmly claim that eating a healthy diet will really prevent cancer after all. We have theories, pathways, mechanisms of action, animal studies, test-tube studies, and studies that look at how people live and eat, but we still aren't at a spot where we can say you will prevent a cancer diagnosis if you eat the way your doctor tells you and take certain supplements.

Sometimes, although not often, someone prefers another product on the pharmacy shelf other than the one I have recommended. This is fine, but in that case, I go into "is this product safe for this patient" mode. As long as there are no disease or drug interactions, then I can rest easier.

As a summary of this chapter, here is a table that reflects the studies showing a benefit from a few given foods as they relate to various types of cancer:

Foods	Participants	Cancer Type	Risk Reduction
Cruciferous vegetables	47,909 4,309 29,361	Bladder Lung Prostate	50% 30% 50%
Tomatoes	47,365	Prostate	25%
Citrus Fruit	521,457	Stomach, Esophagus	25%
Leafy greens (Dietary Folic Acid)	81,922 11,699	Pancreas Breast (post-menopause)	75% 44%
Lignans (flax seeds and others)	58,049	Breast (post-menopause, estrogen-receptor +)	28%
Carrots	470,802	Head and neck	46%
Apples, pears, plums	470,802	Head and neck	38%
Green Tea	69,710	Colorectal	57%
Vegetable oils & Nuts (Dietary tocopherols)	295,344	Prostate	32%
Vitamin D / Calcium	10,578	Breast (pre-menopause)	35%

Source: Béliveau, Gingras, Blaslyk, *Eating Well, Living Well: An Everyday Guide for Optimum Health.*

Regardless of my conclusions about any supplement, I am always happy when the products I offer foster a healthy discussion. Having been a pharmacist for so long, I have worked with many people who have dealt with cancer, so I want to finish this chapter with two brief discussions that I wish I could have with any cancer patient.

All cancers and all cancer patients cannot be painted with the same brush. Patients with advanced stage or metastasized cancer have enormous challenges in maintaining adequate nutrition. Decreased survival time is often seen with a hospitalized cancer patient experiencing more severe malnutrition. Unfortunately, nutrition counseling is not standard therapy for cancer patients, either upon diagnosis or during treatments. This is unfortunate, as cachexia – a wasting of bone and muscle – is common in these patients. Cachexia is secondary to the cancer and is related to a negative energy balance due to the fact that the patient is not hungry or interested in food at any time.

This makes nutrition in cancer patients even more of a challenge, as do nausea, dry mouth, fatigue, dysphagia, constipation, and diarrhea. One way to overcome cachexia or general lack of appetite is through a nutrient-dense food like a broth that brings nutrients back to the body in a dense form. A nutrient-dense broth like the one below provides easily digestible nutrition and reduces side effects like those just mentioned. This type of mixture is relatively easy to make by a family member at home. There are countless ways to do this. Here is one example:

Recipe for Nutritious Broth

- 6 unpeeled carrots, cut into thirds
- 2 unpeeled yellow onions, cut into chunks
- 1 leek, white and green parts, cut into thirds
- 1 bunch celery, including the heart, cut into thirds
- 4 unpeeled red potatoes, quartered

- 2 unpeeled Japanese or regular sweet potatoes, quartered
- 1 unpeeled garnet yam, quartered
- 5 unpeeled cloves of garlic, halved
- One-half bunch of fresh flat-leaf parsley
- One 8-inch strip of kombu (a type of dried seaweed)
- 12 black peppercorns
- 4 whole allspice or juniper berries
- 2 bay leaves
- 8 quarts cold filtered water
- 1 teaspoon sea salt

Instructions:

Rinse the vegetables well, including the kombu. In a 12-quart (or larger) stockpot, combine all ingredients except salt. Fill the pot with water to two inches below the rim, cover, and bring to a boil. Remove the lid; reduce heat to low; and simmer, uncovered, for at least two hours. Add more water if needed to keep vegetables covered. Simmer until the full richness of the vegetables can be tasted. Strain through a large, coarse mesh sieve. Add salt to taste. Let cool to room temperature before refrigerating or freezing.

As a patient progresses to the point of days or weeks to live (negative changes in the patient daily or weekly), the chance of dying of malnutrition before the patient actually succumbs to the disease is less of an issue. Often, family members equate food with love and caring and may not realize that pushing nutrition and fluids at this time can do more harm than good. Realizing that the patient is not hungry and picking up cues like fluid retention and lack of specific organ activity should all be the job of a hospice team. That team should convey to the family that it is time to stop trying to administer nutrition. It is important to closely monitor the palliative patient for the transition in time between when nutrition keeps the patient comfortable and when it causes an overload that the patient cannot handle without distress.

(Stokowski, LA. RN MS. Extreme Nutrition: Can It Beat Cancer? *Medscape Pharmacists.* Nov 20, 2013)

Thoughts on "Big Pharma"

It is common for the average person to be skeptical when it comes to "big pharma" – major multinational pharmaceutical companies. It is not uncommon to hear someone claim that pharmaceutical companies are trying to suppress the real cure for cancer because it would mean their profits would drop off from those sick with cancer. A palliative care doctor in my area once said to me that family members of those pharma executives also get cancer. You would think they would want a cure revealed as well. I personally think that if a cure for cancer (all types) were found, it would be worth trillions of dollars on its own.

Between 2009 and 2013, there were 48 cancer drugs approved by the European Medicines Agency used as treatment for 68 different situations. (Davis C et al. Availability of Evidence of Benefits on Overall Survival and Quality of Life of Cancer Drugs Approved by European Medicines Agency: Retrospective Cohort Study of Drug Approvals 2009-2013. *BMJ.* 2017; 359)

This can be equally dangerous because positive anecdotal evidence is advertised more per incident than those from scientific study. These anecdotal reports have no rigorous statistical testing done to prove if the outcome was a product of chance or not.

HEALTHY LOGIC

CHAPTER 9

ARTHRITIS

"I don't deserve this award,
but I have arthritis and I don't
deserve that either."

– JACK BENNY

First off, arthritis is a catchall phrase that relates to joint pain. There are over one hundred types of arthritis. The most common we see as pharmacists is osteoarthritis, a degenerative joint condition that results from age, infection, or injury to a joint.

Other types of arthritis are autoimmune in nature, meaning they have their origins in your immune system mounting a response against you. Rheumatoid arthritis, psoriatic arthritis, ankylosing spondylitis, and juvenile arthritis are the common types of autoimmune arthritis disorders you may have heard of.

Gout is another form of arthritis. So as you can see, this one term can have many different causes and pathways. Some forms have shown to be genetic in nature. This doesn't mean it's a given that someone will get it, just that the potential is in their DNA. Each of these different types of arthritis also requires different treatments.

Why include a chapter on arthritis? With such intertwined, aging-related subjects like inflammation, immune function, obesity, cardiovascular disease, and pain, why single out this one affliction?

One of the single biggest manifestations of aging decline is the inability to move. Being able to effectively treat a condition that results in reduced mobility is important because mobility equates with healthy aging.

In 2012, *The Lancet* revealed a remarkable analysis on global mortality based on data from 122 countries' individual self-reporting of their lifestyle activity and compared it to overall mortality. Entitled "Effect of Physical Inactivity on Major Non-Communicable Diseases Worldwide: An Analysis of Burden of Disease and Life Expectancy" (Lee IM. *Lancet.* 2012 Jul 21: 380[9838]: 219-29), this analysis states that 9% of premature mortality is caused by inactivity. This is more than 5.3 million of the global total 57 million deaths that occurred in 2008, the year the study data was collected. Like smoking and obesity, sitting and inactivity are now recognized risk factors for mortality.

Complete pain relief in arthritis is seldom achieved, and just because some degree of pain relief is reached, this does not necessarily equate with a drop in associated inflammation or damage.

In pharmacy, when we look at chronic pain, complete pain relief is not a concept we entertain. As always, the patient should be consulted as to what they would like to see as a treatment outcome. I have had some patients completely happy as long as they are able to sleep and are symptom-free enough to make it to church on the weekend. Knowing personal expectations like this is important for the clinician in making a treatment plan. It recognizes that treatment for patients changes as the daily goals of the patients change.

Arthritis can be associated with other conditions, such as lack of sleep, mood disorders like depression, and general fatigue. It can also result in lost wages, lower income, lost time with family, and a decrease in leisure activities such as travel, sports, and hobbies that provide us with mental distance from work and illness. Treating arthritis and the related conditions – or at least being mindful of their presence – is important in having an effect on overall aging.

So, is improving arthritis symptoms and controlling it a benefit to healthy aging? Of course it is! But how do you get control of something that makes moving so painful that you go from being physically active every day to not wanting to move at all?

In the prescription world that I work in, there is no drug or single act that can improve multiple markers like blood cholesterol, glucose, joint mobility, and mood as well as exercise does. Arthritis sees heavy-duty treatments and exciting cutting-edge biologics with promising results. With some of these treatments, benefits can be amazing, although side effects can be strong as well. As with most conditions requiring strong pain relief, physicians are being cautioned more and more to rethink the long-term use of narcotics in non-palliative pain treatment, due to the potential for addiction. However, while this well-intentioned plan is certainly important in fighting the opioid crisis, in the end, with little to replace it for now, opioids will remain in our toolkit.

As healthcare practitioners, we simply have a newfound respect for opioids as new information refines our prescribing habits. We will address this more in the pain chapter, along with other treatments like compounded medications applied through the skin that take the load of oral medications away from the patient.

I have done many talks for different groups on the topic of arthritis, and the number one question is always what they can do to improve symptoms in a non-prescription way. Usually, these inquiries involve glucosamine and chondroitin, the two most popular supplements for arthritis. Sometimes people ask about a product called methylsulfonylmethane, or MSM. As with most nutraceuticals, the problem in determining efficacy or comparing products is the lack of standardization among preparations of the product that hide the actual value (or lack of) that are available to the public.

For osteoarthritis, the "wear and tear, joint breakdown, nonimmune" type of arthritis, which is less inflammatory than rheumatoid arthritis, there is an interesting study called the GAIT Trial (Glucosamine/Chondroitin Arthritis Intervention Trial).

The GAIT Trials were a 2006 US National Institute of Health multimillion-dollar group of studies that tried to determine the efficacy of glucosamine and chondroitin.

The trials have been criticized for several reasons. They included a small number of test patients and funding from commercial sources that supplied the supplements. On top of these problems, the trials had improper blinding of the study (which is crucial for unbiased results). There was also an incredibly high rate of placebo response in this area (upward of 60%), and the relatively mild knee pain in the test subjects with osteoarthritis may have made it difficult to detect a benefit in the treatment groups. Having said this, the authors of the study did do a good job of acknowledging shortcomings of the trial.

The trials looked at glucosamine HCl (500 mg three times daily) and chondroitin sulfate (400 mg three times daily) individually, as well as combined, and compared them with the effect of a positive control, a common prescription medication, celecoxib (200 mg daily), as well as an inactive placebo.

In a conflict of interest, some of the researchers had previous financial ties to the maker of celecoxib. This is a red flag in any study. Another issue is the choice of glucosamine. The HCl form hasn't had the promising results that the sulfate has demonstrated.

The key finding is that the individual or combined ingredients of glucosamine and chondroitin had no benefit on mild to moderate osteoarthritis. The two compounds did, however, show some benefit as a combined therapy in moderate to severe osteoarthritis.

Unfortunately, the two follow-up studies cast doubt on this conclusion. A significant underreported finding in this study was the fact that celecoxib failed to perform better than placebo for any level of osteoarthritis.

Overall, this study seemed to conclude the ineffectiveness of the supplements it was testing, even though the results seemed to suggest otherwise.

In a Cochrane review of 43 randomized controlled trials with nearly 5000 people, chondroitin studies were looked at in people who had osteoarthritis of the knee, hip, and hand. Chondroitin was found to be of some benefit, although the studies were often of low quality.

(http://onlinelibrary.wiley.com/doi/10.1002/14651858. CD005614.pub2/full)

The GUIDE study (Glucosamine Unum-in-Die [once a day] Efficacy) used a 1500 mg daily dose of glucosamine and 3,000 mg acetaminophen in a 24-week study using a placebo as a control. It determined that glucosamine sulfate was a highly cost-effective therapy compared to acetaminophen and placebo for knee osteoarthritis.

A quick search of MSM (methylsulfonylmethane) will give a dog's breakfast of positive, negative, and mixed results on this supplement and its use in treating arthritis. It is an organic sulfur compound that is often used alone or in combination with glucosamine and chondroitin. In one short trial of twelve weeks, subjects (men from 40 to 76 years of age with osteoarthritis of the knee) were given 3 g of MSM, and the experimenters determined that there was an improvement over placebo in the treatment group in both pain reduction and physical function.

(Kim LS, Axelrod LJ, Howard P, Buratovich N, Waters RF. Efficacy of methylsulfonylmethane [MSM] in osteoarthritis pain of the knee: a pilot clinical trial. *Osteoarthritis Cartilage.* 2006 Mar;14[3]: 286-94. Epub 2005 Nov 23.)

Another review, which took place in 2008 and examined both MSM and DMSO (dimethyl sulfoxide) for arthritis, found that DMSO was not proven to aid in osteoarthritis. Although the results of the MSM studies showed positive results, more study is needed to give definitive results on the power of MSM over placebo for osteoarthritis of the knee.

To be fair, all trials with these supplements are not positive in their conclusions. In reviewing what is normally the more promising glucosamine sulfate supplement, seven out of thirteen randomized controlled trials found that this supplement was significantly better than placebo in relieving pain of osteoarthritis, and that side effects were similar to placebo in all thirteen of the reviewed trials. In three out of five trials, there was improvement in walking and other daily activities over placebo with the glucosamine sulfate; however, none of the trials seemed to show a benefit in all symptoms of pain, disability, and stiffness. In fact, it appeared that the more stringent trials were more likely to not determine a benefit from glucosamine.

(Towheed T, Maxwell L, Anastassiades TP, Shea B, Houpt J, RobinsonV et al. Glucosamine therapy for treating osteoarthritis. *Cochrane Database Systematic Review* 2005; 18[2]: CD002946)

(http://www.arthritisresearchuk.org/news/general-news/2012/ july/omega3-fatty-acids-may-reduce-need-for-nsaids-in-rheumatoid-arthritis.aspx)

The Cochrane database reviewed extensively the available evidence for topical anti-inflammatory medications (NSAIDS) and found that ketoprofen and diclofenac were effective topically for osteoarthritis pain, with very little in the way of side effects. The authors of this study endorsed ketoprofen over diclofenac in the area of effectiveness and side effects. (http://onlinelibrary.wiley.com/doi/10.1002/14651858.CD007400.pub3/full)

More on this type of drug will be included in the pain/compounding chapter. Topical and transdermal medications have shown to be of powerful benefit in arthritis pain, with very little in the way of side effects.

ARTHRITIS AND NUTRACEUTICALS

What else does wading into the shark-infested waters of nutraceuticals get us when it comes to relief from arthritis? There are some other useful supplements that have been proven by trials to help:

SAMe

Also known as S-adenosylmethionine, this chemical is found naturally in the body. (Imagine a chemical found naturally in the body! It really does happen.) It is relatively safe, but side effects are magnified in those who are described as "over methylators," since SAMe is a known methyl doner.

Methylation is an important biochemical pathway in our bodies. Adequate methylation pathways are important for gene expression and autoimmune disease. It is also slowly becoming clear that the intestinal microbiome is important in production of methyl donor nutrients. This helps to show why proper gut bacteria is important, not only to your immune system and pain, but also to your mood.

Getting back to arthritis, SAMe was reviewed in a 2002 article that looked at eleven trials that involved this rarely used supplement for arthritis. It found that SAMe was significantly better than placebo and similar to NSAIDs in reducing functional limitations caused by osteoarthritis. It also had a pain-relieving effect similar to NSAIDs and superior to placebo. When the data was reanalyzed from these studies, SAMe patients were found to be 58% less likely to experience side effects than patients on NSAIDs. (Soeken KL, Lee WL, Bausell RB, Agelli M, Berman BM. Safety and efficacy of S-adenosylmethionine (SAMe) for osteoarthritis. *Journal of Family Practice* 2002; 51[5]: 425-30)

In comparing SAMe to celecoxib for osteoarthritis, a 16-week, 2004 trial found that, although it took SAMe longer to work, it was as effective as celecoxib in pain relief and physical function. (Najm WI, Reinsch S, Hoehler F, Tobis JS, Harvey PW. S-adenosylmethionine [SAMe] versus celecoxib for the treatment of osteoarthritis symptoms: a double-blind crossover trial. *BMC Musculoskeletal Disorders* 2004; 26: 5-6)

SAMe isn't recommended, however, if you are on antidepressants, tramadol, or levodopa. Overall, this supplement is surprisingly effective in studies but rarely used as a treatment for osteoarthritis.

OMEGA-3

Turning to one of my personal favourites, omega-3. Studies may not show as much benefit for osteoarthritis as rheumatoid arthritis, but the biochemical pathway that omega-3 follows is the same as the NSAIDs that we give for pain. A confounding factor with most supplement studies is the standardization of what the subjects in each study are taking, and whether or not the conclusions can be extrapolated to represent all supplements with that name on it. The same is true of Omega-3 supplements.

One trial that included 97 people with rheumatoid arthritis had them ingesting fish oil over the course of nine months. A key point to remember here is that most studies with fish oil will test with very low amounts of EPA/DHA, the active ingredients in the oil.

Patients in this study took ten capsules daily of 1 g of oil each, which typically can have anywhere from 300 to 500 mg of EPA/DHA. For arthritis relief, this is the range you need to be into in order to get a noticeable effect. Unfortunately, this may have been the reason for the high rate of dropout in this study (65% of treatment group as opposed to 54% of placebo group), as side effects, mainly gastrointestinal in nature, may have outweighed benefits. Further, a statistically significant 39% of the treatment group reported a reduction in their daily NSAID need (compared to just 10% of the placebo group). This study used a combination of fish liver oil from pressed fish livers and fish body oil from fatty fish tissue, which makes exact conclusions a little murky as to which oil caused the effect. (Galarraga B, Ho M, Youssef HM, Hill A, McMahon H, Hall C, et al. Cod liver oil [n-3 fatty acids] as a non-steroidal anti-inflammatory drug sparing agent in rheumatoid arthritis. *Rheumatology* [Oxford]. 2008; 47[5]: 665–69.)

A review article that focused on just the fish body oil in doses ranging from 1.6 to 7.1 g of omega-3 found that this type of supplement was generally well tolerated and significantly lowered not only joint pain and duration of morning stiffness and fatigue but also reduced the number of painkillers taken per day.

(Fortin PR, Lew RA, Liang MH. Validation of a meta-analysis: the effects of fish oil in rheumatoid arthritis. *Journal of Clinical Epidemiology.* 1995; 48[1]): 1379–90)

As those with rheumatoid arthritis are at an increased risk of cardiovascular disease, it is important to note a long-term study that involved the use of fish oil over a three-year period in those with early rheumatoid arthritis. It concluded that cardiovascular risk was indeed reduced in these patients. (Cleland LG, Caughey GE, James MJ, Proudman SM. Reduction of cardiovascular risk factors with long-term fish oil treatment in early rheumatoid arthritis. *Journal of Rheumatology*. 2006; 33[10]: 1973–79) Unfortunately, a later study that looked at several omega-3 studies found little to no benefit with omega-3 supplementation and cardiovascular outcomes. It is important to note that the effect of omega-3 on arthritic pain can be easier to prove than a longer-term study on omega-3 and cardiovascular health.

Again, results in osteoarthritis with omega-3 are not always promising. Other sources of omega-3 like krill oil and green-lipped mussel from New Zealand need more study. The amount of omega-3 in krill tends to be lower but may be absorbed better than omega-3 contributed from other life-forms. The green-lipped mussel results are a bit more confusing in that it appears to help patients with osteoarthritis when taken with doses of acetaminophen, but there hasn't been much luck in the area of rheumatoid arthritis. All but one study was no better than placebo for this arthritis.

Given the mixed findings on fish oil and the lack of increase in pain relief at increased doses, I recommend food-based sources in a patient's diet first, but most are okay to supplement if they want. It can add up financially to supplement with a good quality omega-3 oil, but I believe it is worth the try, given the risk-benefit analysis of reduced mobility and prescription drug side effects in a long-term use scenario.

The one group of patients I watch for in omega-3 supplementation is anyone on warfarin. Increased bruising or bleeding can occur with even small doses of fish oil and those with a variable INR reading. Bruising or increased bleeding is not uncommon in patients on warfarin when they supplement with even small amounts of fish oil.

OTHER TREATMENTS FOR ARTHRITIS

There are a whole host of supplements, nutraceuticals, and herbs that people use regularly for arthritis. Some of them fall under the heading of "need more information," even though there is anecdotal information about them from patients. Patients contact me for my opinion on a vast array of treatments, including the proteolytic pineapple enzyme known as bromelain, cat's claw, stinging nettle, turmeric, curcumin, willow bark, hydrotherapy, homeopathy, and acupuncture.

There is little doubt that anyone who reads this will have heard a story from someone who swears that one of these has worked and is continuing to work for them. Maybe it even did work for them. The biggest and most legitimate argument from a skeptic or a realist would be the placebo effect, which is especially strong in pain relief.

The key, as always, is to know what is safe and what is not. To be quite honest, virtually all of the glucosamine, chondroitin, and MSM supplements I sell are to people who come into my pharmacy looking for them, not because I have made a recommendation. Some are even looking for help for their dog. Am I confident it will work for them? Based on available science, there is a good chance it will work.

There is an emerging concept in rheumatoid arthritis medication that suggests electrical stimulation of the spleen, which is an important organ in the immune system. You will recall that rheumatoid arthritis is an autoimmune disorder.

The vagus nerve has wide-ranging effects on the body, but when the branch to the spleen is stimulated, it decreases the production of cytokines such as TNF and interleukins, which we mentioned in the inflammation chapter. While the concept of immune regulation in treating rheumatoid arthritis is not new (an expensive group of medications called "biologics" has been doing this for a while), the act of having a direct, non-drug effect on the immune system through the electrical stimulation of one of its organs is innovative.

Or is it? Proponents of acupuncture and chiropractic have leaped on this electrical stimulation idea and are claiming that they have been doing this all along. This connection between improving the immune system and acupuncture certainly needs more study before someone like myself would say there is a connection. In regard to acupuncture, there appears to be some immune system activity, but proof in studies appears inconsistent.

(Arranz L1, Guayerbas N, Siboni L, De la Fuente M. Effect of acupuncture treatment on the immune function impairment found in anxious women. *Am J Chin Med.* 2007; 35(1): 35-51)

In eight Cochrane reviews of studies for various pain disorders, acupuncture was found to be effective for peripheral joint osteoarthritis. (Lee MS et al. *Chin J Integr Med.* 2011 Mar;17(3): 187-9) Further, Cochrane reviews reveal that although the results of placebo-controlled trials are statistically significant, the benefit seems to be small and may not reach clinical relevance. I am often asked my opinion of acupuncture on the treatment of many symptoms. For the effectiveness of using acupuncture to treat arthritis, it would be difficult to find a doctor who hasn't heard a success story anecdotally from one or more of their patients. I have heard the same. I could produce an equal number of trials either for or against acupuncture for arthritis. Whether acupuncture has any clinically significant effects depends on who you ask. Again, safety first, efficacy second dictates that if someone is getting a perceived benefit from something and the treatment is safe, there should be no problem, but hard evidence is lacking.

Now, if someone is getting their neck adjusted at the chiropractor, the safety aspect comes into play, not to mention the effectiveness as well. Most physicians I speak to would encourage the patient to pursue acupuncture if they felt it was working for them, regardless of the evidence for or against it. As far as chiropractic adjustments affecting the immune system in any way though, there is zero evidence for this.

As far as non-pharmacological treatment of arthritis-associated fatigue, there is a proven benefit in regular physical activity and psychosocial interventions such as a support network, outreach services, and needs management. (http://onlinelibrary.wiley.com/doi/10.1002/14651858.CD011338/full)

These findings are repeated over and over again in many disease prevention and treatment regimens. (http://onlinelibrary.wiley.com/doi/10.1002/14651858.CD010538/full)

Some lesser-known therapies that have been found clinically to improve joint health and reduce pain include a product called iso-alpha acids, which is often derived from hops. These inhibit what is called kinase activity in the joints.

A few years ago, I attended a conference on pain at Dalhousie University in Halifax. Kinase activity was presented in detail there as a novel approach to relieving pain in joints. Dealing with kinase activity avoided the gastrointestinal and cardiovascular side effects of NSAIDs in rheumatoid arthritis. It is a fascinating world treatment that targets joints via the immune system. As an added benefit, products that contain these types of compounds are available over the counter. Prescription agents are now available that inhibit kinase enzymes and prevent the release of mediators called cytokines that stimulate inflammation in rheumatoid arthritis. There are also other pathways used by prescription medications to prevent inflammation that involve tumour necrosis factor (TNF) and interleukin-6 (IL-6), as well as selective T cell activity. The immune system pathways have proven very effective in bringing medications to market for rheumatoid arthritis.

(Konda VR, Desai A, Darland G, Bland JS, Tripp ML. Rho iso-alpha acids from hops inhibit the GSK-3/NF-⬛B pathway and reduce inflammatory markers associated with bone and cartilage degradation. *Journal of Inflammation* [London, England]. 2009; 6:26. DOI:10.1186/1476-9255-6-26)

VITAMIN D

What about vitamin D? You can find many studies and stories that correlate low vitamin D with a whole myriad of disease states. There are now a growing number of studies that show that supplementing a patient with rheumatoid arthritis who is low in vitamin D can help improve the disease. (http://www.ncbi.nlm.nih.gov/pubmed/26481198) It also turns out these patients are often low in vitamin D anyway, even though not deficient – not surprising. A second study verified that disease severity was higher with persons that had lower vitamin D; however, when the low vitamin D patients were supplemented with the vitamin, there wasn't a statistically significant difference in their flare-ups. It is generally recognized that vitamin D supplementation plays some sort of a role in autoimmune disease and pain relief, but the lack of continuity among trials and the lack of such trials leaves this question unanswered. (Leventis P, Patel S. Clinical aspects of vitamin D in the management of rheumatoid arthritis. *Rheumatology.* 2008. 47 [11]: 1617-1621. First published online August 5, 2008)

The take-home message is that there is no harm in taking a blood test to see if your level of vitamin D needs supplementation to bring it back into normal ranges and to measure the effect that might have on arthritic pain. Vitamin D is a relatively inexpensive supplement that may be low anyway, especially in the senior North American population, who may not get adequate sun exposure. (Yang J1, Liu L1, Zhang Q2, Li M1, Wang J. Effect of vitamin D on the recurrence rate of rheumatoid arthritis. *Exp Ther Med.* 2015 Nov;10[5]: 1812-1816. Epub 2015 Sep 15)

In conclusion, we know that low vitamin D is a risk factor in arthritis flare-ups, but we are just a little less clear on the effect of supplementing D.

It is important to keep in mind the reason that we are trying to improve arthritis symptoms in the first place, which is to help prolong life by increasing movement.

OTHER PROMISING NATURAL SUPPLEMENTS FOR JOINT PAIN

Natural Eggshell Membrane: 500 mg taken once daily has shown evidence for pain relief. (*Clin Rheumatol.* 2009 Aug; 28[8]: 907-914)

Serrapeptidase is widely used and has been studied for pain relief with some promising results, but the evidence is not quite there to recommend this for pain relief. (Bhagat S, Agarwal M, Roy V. Serratiopeptidase: A systematic review of the existing evidence. *International Journal of Surgery* [London, England]. 2013. 11. 10.1016 / j.ijsu.2013.01.010)

Boswellia serrate has been shown in small studies to work for osteoarthritis of the knee (Kimmatkar N1, Thawani V, Hingorani L, Khiyani R. Efficacy and tolerability of Boswellia serrata extract in treatment of osteoarthritis of knee – a randomized double-blind placebo-controlled trial. *Phytomedicine.* 2003 Jan;10[1]: 3-7)

Devil's claw has also been used, although good studies are lacking on both efficacy and long-term safety, and **curcumin** is a favourite pain relief compound that has also been studied. Although evidence isn't strong enough for pharmacists to recommend curcumin for pain relief right now, there is compelling evidence to include this dietary supplement as an add-on ingredient to conventional therapy. Curcumin is typically not absorbed well, leading to very expensive supplements that have been modified to increase absorption.

All of these supplements have been studied and all have proposed mechanisms for pain and or inflammation, especially in joints. This means that we have a possible pathway of how they all may work. However, it is important to separate this from the claim that each one works. Talk to your pharmacist for more information on using these supplements.

HEALTHY LOGIC

CHAPTER 10

PERSONAL CLINICAL EXPERIENCE

"Statistical results with a causal interpretation have a stronger effect on our thinking than non-causal information. But even compelling causal statistics will not change long-held beliefs or beliefs rooted in personal experience."

– DANIEL KAHNEMAN

Sifting through studies with both positive and negative outcomes gives us a solid foundation with which to make our own decisions on whether or not to try a therapy on our own. Certainly, when I am making recommendations, this is what I do. To simply refer to an opinion by Health Canada or a position statement from a pharmaceutical group may be helpful, but in the end, I often feel that my patients deserve more due diligence than that.

In my clinical experience, there are some clear hits and misses that stand out. In science, we always aspire for a clear yes or no answer, but in many cases I feel the public is better served by categorizing some products as "promising." This either means keep an eye out for future developments or at least that they aren't totally off the wall; and a lot of the over-the-counter world really is off the wall. No one hears more than a pharmacist how many people will only take something that is "natural" or "plant-based." In the world of natural products, I often find myself pointing out the fact that over 120 conventional pharmaceutical products are derived from plant species. (http://www.uptodate.com/contents/overview-of-herbal-medicine-and-dietary-supplements)

What follows here is a brief summary of which supplements I feel work and which don't work. As is the case for this entire book, there is zero influence by any group, individual, or company, monetary or otherwise, in making these recommendations. Although there are a number of specific brands I use with success and are my "go-to" treatments, I am leaving them out of this discussion to avoid any impression of support for any third party. Please note that personal belief is not science – going with evidence is science. There are, however, many products in the OTC section that haven't been explored fully, and it is not uncommon for prescribers and pharmacists to rely on patient feedback and clinical experience in their recommendations. As always, don't go on any supplement without speaking to your healthcare professional.

When you ask for a pharmacist's advice, understanding a patient's symptoms and making a recommendation that contributes to a measurable improvement in their quality of life is our goal. Please note that these recommendations represent a snapshot in time. I will be classifying each product as either a hard "miss" (don't bother) or a "hit" (try it), so this process leaves room for the odd reader who disagrees based on their personal experience. I do not disregard anyone's experience; I am simply relating my own.

GINKGO BILOBA FOR MEMORY – MISS

Anyone in the supplement world is familiar with ginkgo. Regardless of what I have read in studies, I really have never seen this herb do much benefit. One promising use I had hope for and followed a few studies on was with vertigo, a major problem for many people that can be quite debilitating. Although long-term use may be needed for a benefit, it never seemed to pan out for anyone I've seen use it. Improved memory is another major claim by many products with ginkgo. Again, I have never seen much benefit. In truth, it is not something I have ever recommended. (http://www.ncbi. nlm.nih.gov/pubmed/23001963; http://www.ncbi.nlm.nih.gov/pubmed/11026748)

OMEGA-3 FOR PAIN – HIT

With the growing awareness that oral NSAIDS are not safe to take long term, especially in seniors, an alternative pain reliever for general pain, such as that found in arthritis, is often sought after. Acetaminophen is often used for this reason; however, in doses I am seeing, less acetaminophen would be preferred. The daily load on the liver by this medication is relentless, and the lack of anti-inflammatory action by it leaves a patient undertreated in some cases. I have seen lives changed by Omega-3 supplementation, especially when a high-quality supplement is given at a sufficient dose (at least 4 g of combined EPA/DHA per day). Some physicians are using this instead of NSAIDS for back pain. Just be careful if you are on a blood thinner because your bleeding times or bruising may increase.

KRILL OIL – HIT

Virtually the same as omega-3 for benefits, but the EPA and DHA are altered in a way that increases absorption, so the dose becomes reduced. Studies conclude the same as above, including ability to improve arthritis pain. (http://www.ncbi.nlm.nih.gov/pubmed/17353582)

GLUCOSAMINE WITH OR WITHOUT CHONDROITIN – MISS

Now here's one I wish I could agree with. If there is an alternative therapy that is used by seemingly everyone, this is it. There are those who swear by it. The problem is, there are really no good trials to show that it works for arthritis in any way. A relatively large study followed 600 people over two years in conjunction with a placebo group. There was a slight possibility of a potential benefit, if the results were extrapolated over a 15-year period (in knee replacement avoidance), but the statistical significance of the study was not promising. Personal clinical experience for me isn't nearly consistent enough to recommend it. (http://www.ncbi.nlm.nih.gov/pubmed/24395557)

In a huge study known as GAIT, which we discussed in the arthritis chapter. similar results were determined. (https://nccih.nih.gov/research/results/gait)

So, although there seems to be an inkling of benefit for some arthritis sufferers out there, this is one supplement that is just not worth the money, in my opinion.

HOMEOPATHY – MISS

As much as I would like to see a group of therapies with so few side effects work, I must pass on this one. Obviously, the reason for the low side effect profile of homeopathic medications is the lack of ingredients to cause them in the first place. There is no shortage of practitioners who feel these medications do work, but I'm just not one of them.

VACCINATIONS – HIT

There is no safer treatment for curing diseases in humans than vaccines. I must stress the importance of vaccines and the complete selfishness of not vaccinating. I am certainly pro-vaccination, not only to protect yourself, but to protect the unprotected who are in legitimate danger of contracting disease, like the immunocompromised and infants not yet vaccinated.

HPV VACCINE FOR BOYS AND GIRLS – HIT

Being a relatively new vaccine, this one has attracted its fair share of antivax comments. The safety and efficacy of this vaccine, combined with its proven track record to save lives by decreasing cervical cancer for women and head and neck cancer in men, will continue to grow.

COENZYME Q10 WITH STATINS – MISS

In Chapter 6 on micronutrient deficiencies, we discussed statins. You will recall that statins lower cholesterol and repair the insides of blood vessels. We also mention CoQ10. The effects of CoQ10 depletion are clear as far as negative cardiovascular outcomes go. As a pharmacist, I see statins used daily and am aware of the backlash against this medication because of the side effect profile it has (including a reported increased risk of diabetes and possibly Alzheimer's). At the moment however, statins are the best we have to deal with plaque buildup and rupture. Muscle pain from statins is actually very rare, although some patients come off this drug for this reason. Some feel CoQ10 helps prevent this side effect from happening. Again, not much is available to back this up. The cost involved with taking both the statin and the coenzyme are prohibitive for many patients, so I don't often have the opportunity to observe this combination. It is a terrific concept, and I'd love to say this is a hit, but barring any personal experience to go with, the data says no for the most part. Safe to try, though!

(http://www.uptodate.com/contents/statin-myopathy/abstract/146 and http://www.uptodate.com/contents/statin-myopathy/abstract/147)

PROBIOTICS (WITH OR WITHOUT ANTIBIOTICS) – HIT

The effects of antibiotics on the gut flora are well documented. An unwanted effect of killing off friendly bacteria in the gut by the antibiotic can result in an intestine that doesn't function as it should, resulting in diarrhea. Including probiotics in one's dietary regimen replaces friendly bacteria that has been lost, helping to restore gut function and relieving the diarrhea. As humans, we tend to gravitate toward immediate results, especially when paying out of pocket for something. A well-balanced gut flora has a positive effect on everything from GI function to mental well-being, the immune system, pain relief, and skin inflammation. http://www.uptodate.com/contents/candida-vulvovaginitis/abstract/103

http://www.uptodate.com/contents/prebiotics-and-probiotics-for-treatment-of-allergic-disease/abstract/14

http://www.uptodate.com/contents/prebiotics-and-probiotics-for-treatment-of-allergic-disease/abstract/21

http://www.jpeds.com/article/S0022-3476(04)00634-1/pdf

http://onlinelibrary.wiley.com/doi/10.1002/14651858.CD006895.pub3/abstract

http://www.ncbi.nlm.nih.gov/pmc/articles/PMC2664325/

RELORA FOR ANXIETY – HIT

Intermittent or chronic anxiety can be frustrating to treat, and OTC therapies can be hit or miss at best; however, Relora is, in my opinion, your best bet for attempting a body-friendly way of treating anxiety before jumping to a prescription. (http://www.jissn.com/content/10/1/37 and http://www.ncbi.nlm.nih.gov/pubmed/18426577)

TRIBULUS TERRESTRIS FOR TESTOSTERONE INCREASE – MISS

Although libido may be enhanced in men (at least male rats) as well as erectile function (and even these studies are weak at best), actual testosterone levels shouldn't be expected to rise therapeutically with this supplement.

DETOX – MISS

Again, I need to go with the science here. A full book can be written on this topic and its ongoing debate. The principles of detox sound good on paper. Detox is supposed to help liver pathways to remove toxins, give antioxidant support to protect tissues against free radicals, and biochemically remove what needs to be removed from the body. Detoxes regularly include items that will bind with toxins and metals (chlorella, spirulina, and insoluble fibre – all healthy supplements anyway), and recommend eating lots of greens and drinking lots of water. Quite often detox regimens include healthy things to do anyway. I do not doubt that the above-mentioned dietary choices will make someone feel better, and if they grab and eliminate some bad stuff during the process, then so much the better. There are, however, detoxes that are on the extreme side of the scale that concern me. All juicing detoxes, total starvation, total soup, "total" anything, really. Anything that is all of one thing for too long carries inherent risks, not the least of which is nutrient depletion.

One idea that promoters of detox stress is modern medicine's complete lack of understanding of autoimmune disease. They will claim that removing toxins will help the body to not overreact to toxins, which ostensibly, is what leads to autoimmune disorders.

Anything that touts itself as an aid or stimulant for the liver, sweat glands, lungs, intestines, and kidneys is, in my experience not backed by evidence. In all likelihood, these products will not do more to remove "toxins" than would healthy diet changes.

DIM OR I3C – HIT

I recommend these relatively inexpensive supplements (diindoly-methane and indole-3-carbinol) also found in food, because they keep the 2-hydroxy estrogens up and the 4- and 16-hydroxy estrogens low. The latter estrogens are correlated more closely with cancer than the former. In men, these supplements may also lead to a more favourable testosterone/estrogen balance. Clinically, I have little to show what this will do for a patient disease-wise, however. These compounds are derived from cruciferous vegetables.

If someone is not interested in a supplement and wants to eat healthily, I recommend dietary sources of **glucosinolates**. Below is a list of examples of foods with corresponding amounts of glucosinolates for each. Check with your pharmacist if you are on blood thinners before changing your diet to include more of the cruciferous vegetables listed below. In this list, which includes the glucosinolate levels of various foods, any food that includes diindolylmethane or its precursor, indole-3-carbinol, is bolded:

Brussels Sprouts, 104 mg glucosinolate per 44 g (half cup)
Garden Cress, 98 mg per 25 g (half cup)
Mustard Greens, 79 mg per 28 g (half cup, chopped)
Turnip, 60 mg per 65 g (half cup, cubes)
Savoy Cabbage, 35 mg per 45 g (half cup, chopped)
Kale, 67 mg per 67 g (1 cup, chopped)
Watercress, 32 mg per 34 g (1 cup, chopped)
Kohlrabi, 31 mg per 67 g (half cup, chopped)
Red Cabbage, 29 mg per 45 g (half cup, chopped)
Broccoli, 27 mg per 44 g (half cup, chopped)
Horseradish, 24 mg per 15 g (tablespoon)
Cauliflower, 22 mg per 50 g (half cup chopped)
Bok Choy, 19 mg per 35 g (half cup, chopped)

SULFORAPHANE FOR PROSTATE CANCER PREVENTION – HIT

Many promising studies have been done on this broccoli extract and its potential for benefits with prostate cancer. These recommendations fall under the same strength as the DIM and I3C recommendations above in firm outcomes, but these studies are interesting in the effects of sulforaphane on cancer cell death and testosterone metabolite levels.

http://www.ncbi.nlm.nih.gov/pubmed/11836580
http://www.pnas.org/content/106/39/16663.abstract
http://www.ncbi.nlm.nih.gov/pubmed/25051139
http://www.cancernetwork.com/prostate-cancer/asco-sulforaphane-prostate-cancer-found-worthy-further-investigation
http://www.jbc.org/content/280/20/19911.abstract

ZINC – HIT

The list of clinically proven benefits from this essential mineral is long. Personally, I see immediate benefits in cold, flu, and respiratory tract infections. Many studies show benefits only when one's zinc status is low; however, this is not an uncommon state to be in. Zinc loss occurs with sweating, oral contraceptive use, antacid use (including H2 antagonists and PPIs), ACE inhibitors, NSAIDS, and some diabetic as well as vegetarian diets. Correcting zinc levels helps T4 and T3 levels for your thyroid health and increases sperm count. Zinc can also be an effective treatment for warts (both oral and topical administration). In a few studies, there have been notable positive effects in resistant depression, but only when combined with conventional pharmaceutical therapy.

(http://www.ncbi.nlm.nih.gov/pubmed/19278731) As an aside, this finding is interesting in that zinc interacts with a receptor known as NMDA in the body, as does ketamine, which has shown promise in nasal spray application for depression.

VITAMIN K2 – HIT

The "calcification paradox" of osteoporosis and arterial calcification in menopause is soundly addressed with calcium, vitamin D and vitamin K2 supplementation. The result is even better with hormone replacement therapy (preferably of the bio-identical kind). Vitamin K2 is used by the body to drive calcium to the bones and not to other tissues such as blood vessels and soft tissues, where it is not needed and can cause harm. K2 is now included in some bone-building supplements. There is a caution that it may reduce the effect of warfarin but not necessarily enhance the occurrence of clots in patients. So it is often taken together with a prescriber's permission. (http://www.ncbi.nlm.nih.gov/pubmed/16030366 and

http://www.ncbi.nlm.nih.gov/pubmed/16801507)

THE MEDITERRANEAN DIET – HIT

I am not a dietician, but I know there are many, many healthy ways to eat. If you're keeping an eye on what you eat for weight loss, disease prevention, specific health benefits, or because of a specific disease state or medication, it's best to first seek proper counselling from your healthcare provider. However, if you're just looking for a best practices way to eat, the Mediterranean Diet does hold some weight, especially with regards to cardiovascular health, which is a major health risk for us all. (Martinez-Gonzalez, MA et al. The Mediterranean Diet and Cardiovascular Health. *Circulation Research.* 2019; 124: 779-798)

GARCINIA CAMBOGIA / RASPBERRY KETONES – MISS

I'll lump these two together since they don't deserve any extra room for consideration. They're both fad weight-loss ideas that had a meteoric rise and pretty much just as meteoric a fall. They both fall on the heap of nothing more than fad, and not even safe, supplements. Liver toxicity has been reported with Garcinia Cambogia.

FIBRE – HIT

One of the best proven supplements you can take is fibre. Inflammation caused by constipation is easily one of the most common issues I see as a pharmacist. From hormone health to intestinal health, constipation is treatable with nonabsorbable, and for the most part low side-effect, fibre products. It is easy to obtain sufficient levels of fibre through diet alone, but there are completely safe OTC supplements available. If you want to take a fibre supplement, here are a few simple rules: start slow, drink lots of water, and don't take a dose at the same time as medications. If you only take one supplement, it should be fibre. The Canadian Diabetes Association touts soluble fibre as an effective aid for lowering blood glucose spikes after meals and also as an effective means of keeping cholesterol down. Studies have proven the benefits of increased whole grains in coronary heart disease patients (http://www.ncbi.nlm.nih.gov/pubmed?term=15585760) and in reducing the risk of stroke. (http://www.ncbi.nlm.nih.gov/pubmed?term=7707599

CALCIUM AND VITAMIN D FOR FRACTURE PREVENTION – HIT

For most adults over 50 who are active and eat a well-balanced diet, the best recommendations will always be to get out in the sunshine and to practice yoga, Pilates, Tai Chi, or other balance-enhancing activities that prevent falls. If you are already living by these recommendations, then supplementation probably isn't going to be of much benefit. However, it would not be uncommon to see someone living away from the equator experience a vitamin D slump, and therefore, especially given the low cost of each of these supplements, I list them as a hit.

CELL PHONES AND CANCER – MISS

So far, claims about the negative effects of cell phones on the body should be relegated to the status of "fear-mongering." There have actually been many studies on this topic, both on animals and humans. To help us understand, we go back to the concept of the null hypotheses, which we talked about earlier. It is assumed everything is false until proven true. If statistical analysis says we can say with relative certainty that something is true, then we reject the null hypothesis and say there is a cause-and-effect relationship.

Many robust studies using large numbers of people have consistently shown no cause-and-effect relationship between cell phone use and cancer. People who tell you cell phones cause brain cancer are cherry-picking – choosing studies to back up their point while leaving the others conveniently on the shelf. One study showed an increased cancer rate in rodents who were exposed to intense radiation (not exactly cell phone stuff). Even in that study, many of the rats that were exposed to radiation lived longer than the control rats with no radiation, and therefore had much more time to develop cancer. The consensus is, no increased cancer from cell phones.

FLUORIDE IN DRINKING WATER – HIT

An unproven theory states that fluoride in drinking water acts like iodine and messes with your thyroid. This is a make-believe story that has been making its way around social media for years. This is a topic I bring up from time to time with dentists, and the answer is always the same: although there is a physiological mechanism whereby fluoride can interact with thyroid hormones, the level of fluoridation we typically receive in drinking water and toothpaste has not been found to cause anything clinically significant. (Barberio, AM et al. Fluoride exposure and indicators of thyroid functioning in the Canadian population: implications for community water fluoridation. Correspondence to Dr. Lindsay McLaren, Department of Community Health Sciences and O'Brien Institute for Public Health, University of Calgary)

EXERCISE FOR SUCCESSFUL AGING – HIT

The benefits of exercise should now be obvious to most readers. If you need a study, there are plenty out there, but I will leave you with this one. An Australian study of over 1500 adults over the age of 49 who did not have a history of cancer, stroke, or coronary artery disease were followed for ten years. In measuring markers of aging, the researchers were looking for depression symptoms, cognitive decline, disability, respiratory symptoms, and conditions like cancer and coronary artery disease. Participants who engaged in the highest levels of physical activity compared to the lowest showed a greater likelihood of successfully aging ten years later. (Gopinath B, Kifley A, Flood VM, Mitchell P. Physical Activity as a Determinant of Successful Aging over Ten Years. *Scientific Reports.* 2018. Vol. 8, Article 10522)

CHAPTER 11

PAIN & COMPOUNDING

"No condition gives more
relief when treated sufficiently
to both patient and physician
than chronic pain."

– UNKNOWN AUTHOR

Overall, the number one reason I see for decreased quality of life, lost work time, and increased costs of rehabilitation is pain. If there is one thing we have a problem imaging, running diagnostic tests for, or just putting an objective measurement on, it is pain.

In pharmacy school, we were taught to treat pain with acetaminophen, or, if inflammation is present, ibuprofen, naproxen, or Aspirin over the counter. If treatment with these options fails, then it is followed by yet another NSAID on a prescription, the most common options being higher-strength ibuprofen, naproxen, celecoxib, or ketorolac.

When the higher-strength NSAIDs fail, then we see opioids used: codeine, morphine, hydromorphone, oxycodone, etc. This progression has been the routine for many, many years. It has resulted in an opioid epidemic that has destroyed lives and shattered the public's belief in the pharmaceutical system.

Without a doubt, the single best thing I did regarding my pharmacy business was to introduce compounding. Simply put, compounding is when your pharmacists makes your prescription from scratch rather than taking it from a bottle that has been made in a finished form from a drug company. Compounding opened up a whole world of individualized treatment for the patients in my area.

I had a very good introduction to supplements by a Dr. Frank Chandler at Dalhousie University and worked for a rare compounding pharmacy run by Byron Sarson near the University for the four years I attended pharmacy school. It was an invaluable first exposure to individualized medicine.

Dr. Chandler, the Dean of the Dalhousie College of Pharmacy, taught a course that went through each vitamin, mineral, and herb, and discussed what each one does pharmacologically in the body, as well as its dietary sources, recommended amounts, and just about any other piece of information we would need in counselling the public. Part of this information dealt with the individualized nature of supplements, the reasons why one person is deficient and the next is not, even when they have the same diets, even if they are identical twins. Little did I realize then how much problem this one wall in the pharmacy would give me later on in my pharmacy career. The key learning point was the "individualized" nature of supplements, not just reading the studies on those that are widely taken for prevention and treatment of disease – which is also important.

Byron Sarson was my first boss in pharmacy. He ran a rare compounding pharmacy in Halifax in the late 1980s. Esmonde Cooke, a former dean of the College who retired in my hometown, recommended I speak to Sarson. That's how I started at the job that would influence the rest of my career. Little did I know at the time that individualized medicine would become the norm. I was introduced to a treatment model that most pharmacies didn't have yet. Unavailable meds, discontinued meds, fine-tuned strengths, dosage forms, allergies, adverse-effect avoidance, and other specific problems were all reasons for patients to need our specialized, personalized advice. Compounding became an exciting way to practice pharmacy. Witnessing Byron's problem-solving interactions with his patients was one of the most important learning experiences I had and influences my own patient interactions to this day.

One of Doctor Chandler's points of interest involved omega-3. To believe that omega-3 could actually help for pain? How could that be? This is a claim that I would have glossed over as just another supplement claim in theory back then. Little did I know that it would be one of the most recommended products of mine for pain twenty years after I graduated. Omega-3 works along the same pathway that our regular NSAIDS do for pain. Studies such as this dual-centre, double-blinded, placebo-controlled trial have demonstrated that an omega 3 oil such as cod liver oil helps relieve rheumatoid arthritis pain. (http://www.ncbi.nlm.nih.gov/pubmed/18362100)

There is no shortage of studies on this topic. For those with back pain (unfortunately often referred to as a diagnosis when it's a symptom), omega-3 has shown promise. (http://www.ncbi.nlm.nih.

gov/pubmed/16531187) Also shown in this study is the possibility of reducing or discontinuing NSAIDs for pain, something I see clinically as well.

This study suggests that supplementing with omega-3 not only improved back and neck pain, but it also reduced prescription medication and had no significant side effects. This study was a questionnaire given to 125 patients who reported on their omega-3 use. Of course, this study does not make a clear conclusion, like "Omega-3 Kills Pain." Any study that makes a claim like that is not a study but a marketing document and should be approached with caution. All the same, I believe these results to be interesting.

So, what of the compounding I mentioned earlier in the chapter? Without a doubt, I think the most interesting area in compounding is in transdermal pain relief, particularly in palliative care. Transdermal pain relief involves hitting pain-transmitting nerves at as many different receptors as possible by creating a salve that is applied to the skin.

The types of pain that I treat transdermally are soft tissue pain, shingles-related pain, joint pain, nerve pain, phantom limb pain in amputees, palliative care or oncology-related pain, wound and pressure ulcer pain, and dental-related pain. The most common ingredients used in topical pain relief are common pain relievers, simply applied through a different delivery method. These include various combinations and strengths of amitriptyline, clonidine, gabapentin, ketamine, ketoprofen, lidocaine, diclofenac, morphine, baclofen, cyclobenzaprine, and lorazepam, to name a few.

Studies exist for each of these ingredients, one of my favourite reference guides being "Compounded Pain Formulations, What's the Evidence?" (Scott Asbill et al. *Int J Pharm Compd.* Jul-Aug 2014) A local palliative care and pain physician, Dr. John Ritter, and I have used various combinations of these compounds, which we make from scratch in the compounding lab of the pharmacy. I must stress that these active pharmaceutical ingredients are not something we dreamed up, so we cannot claim any originality on these products. These are compounded at many progressive compounding pharmacies, and I always search out as many studies as possible before an ingredient is included in a salve for one of our patients. In the end, after the research has been completed, it is the success of that ingredient in treating pain that pushes its continuation in our recommendations. John and I have been lucky enough to team up with a chemist from Cape Breton University in Nova Scotia to show the ability of our compounded pain creams to deliver these active pharmaceutical ingredients through the skin and into the tissue.

Here are the results of three different bases with six active ingredients all passing through a synthetic skin substitute at the same time. A follow-up study now being done will compare these results to the originals shown here. We used three commonly used bases for transdermal delivery of drugs through the skin: Salt Stable LS from Humco, Transdermal Pain Base from Medisca, and Lipoderm Activemax from PCCA. Each drug is represented by two graphs. One shows the flux of that active ingredient over time (meaning the flow of the active ingredient through the membrane into the proposed tissue space in the body). The second graph is the cumulative transfer of the active ingredient over time into the space on the other side of the membrane. Put another way, these graphs give a visual representation of what happens to the active ingredient after it is applied to the skin, whether it gets absorbed into the tissue where it can have an effect on a nerve in pain relief, and how much of the drug actually passes through over a given period of time. This was done in order to prove to prescribers as well as patients that what we are giving them is actually passing through tissue to where it needs to be working. Turns out all three commonly used bases for pain creams work well to do what they claim and deliver multiple ingredients to the affected area.

TRANSDERMAL PENETRATION STUDY

2% Amitriptyline + 2% Ketamine + 2% Ketoprofen + 0.02% Clonidine
HCL + 1.2% Gabapentin + 0.4% Lidocaine

Amitriptyline

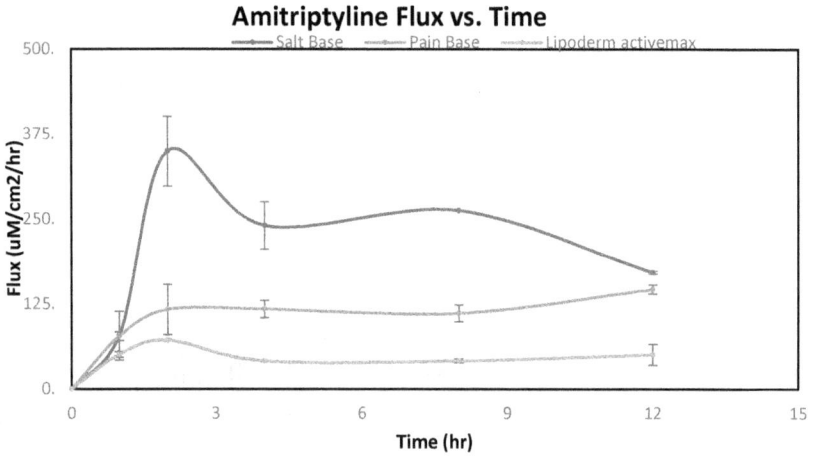

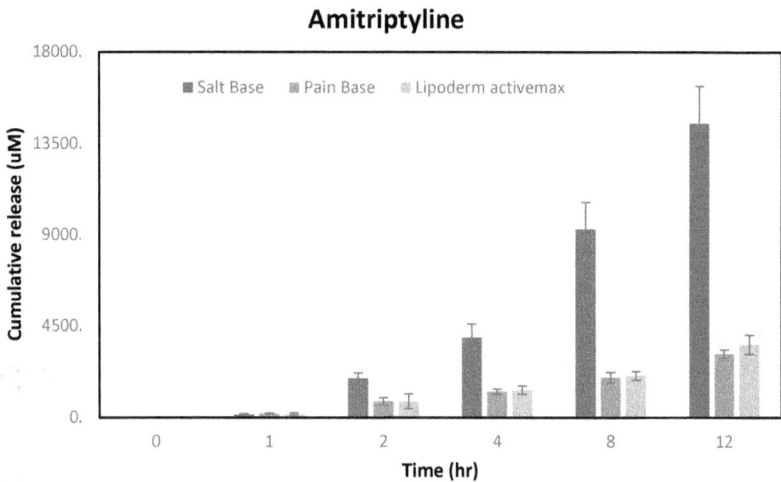

Ketamine

Ketamine

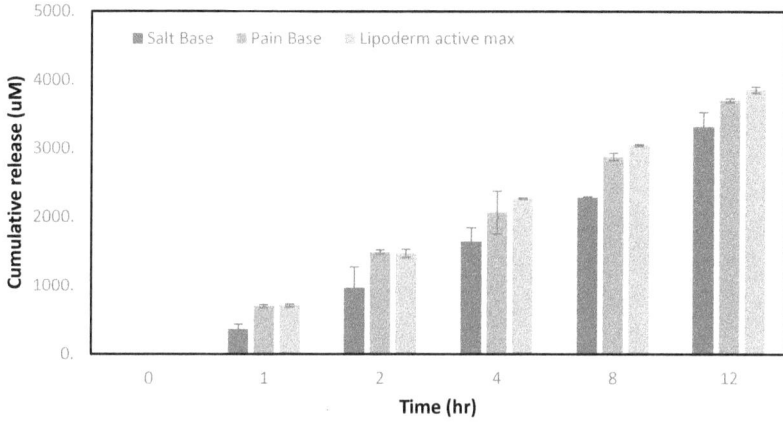

Ketamine Flux vs. Time

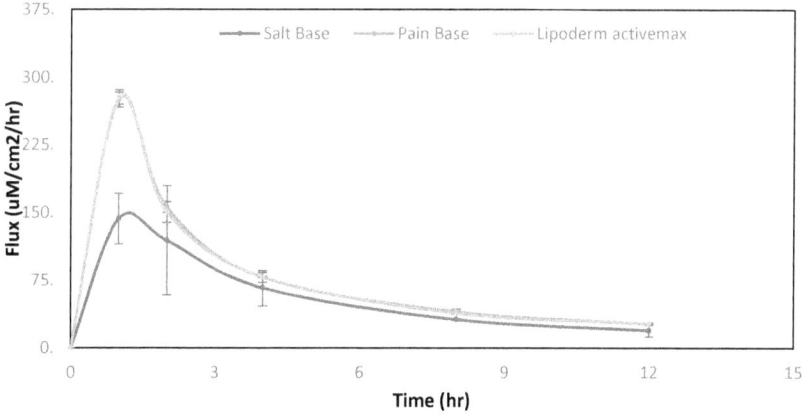

Ketoprofen

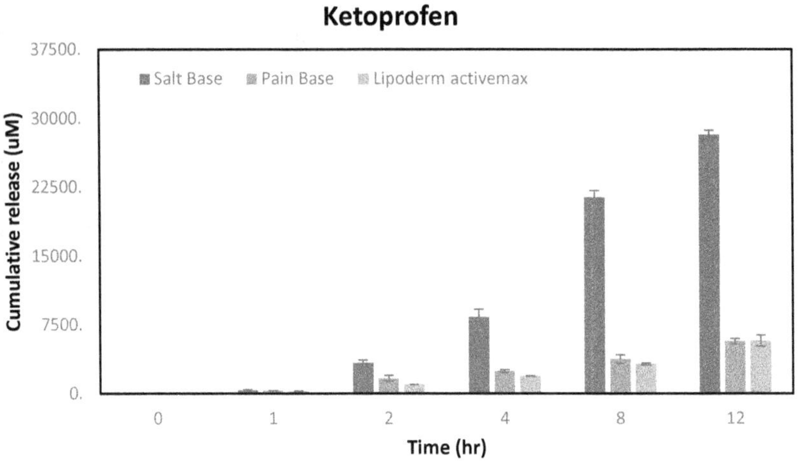

Ketoprofen
Salt Base
Pain Base
Lipoderm activemax
Cumulative release (uM)
37500.
30000.
22500.
15000.
7500.
0.
0
1
2
4
8
12
Time (hr)

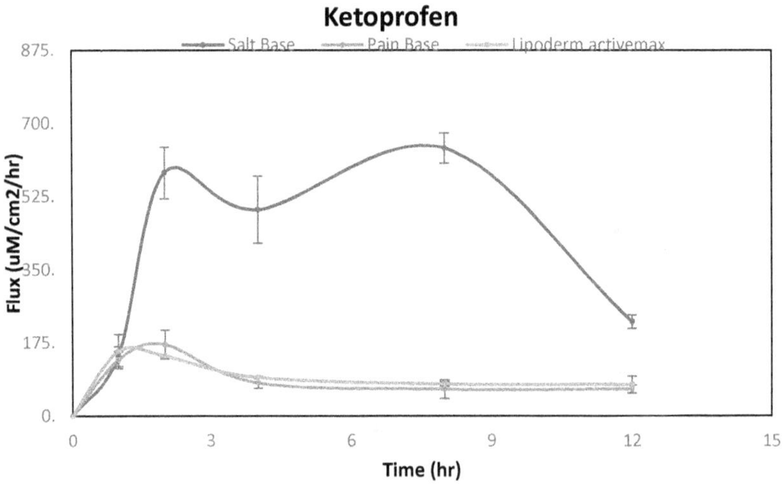

Ketoprofen
Salt Base
Pain Base
Lipoderm activemax
Flux (uM/cm2/hr)
875.
700.
525.
350.
175.
0.
0
3
6
9
12
15
Time (hr)

Clonidine HCL

Clonidine

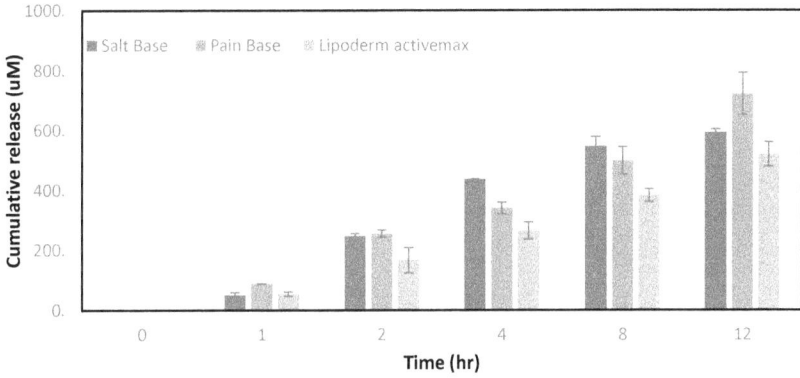

Clonidine Flux vs. Time

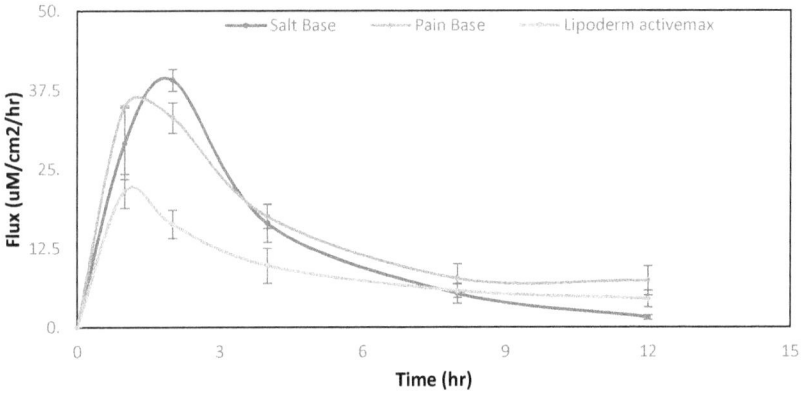

Gabapentin

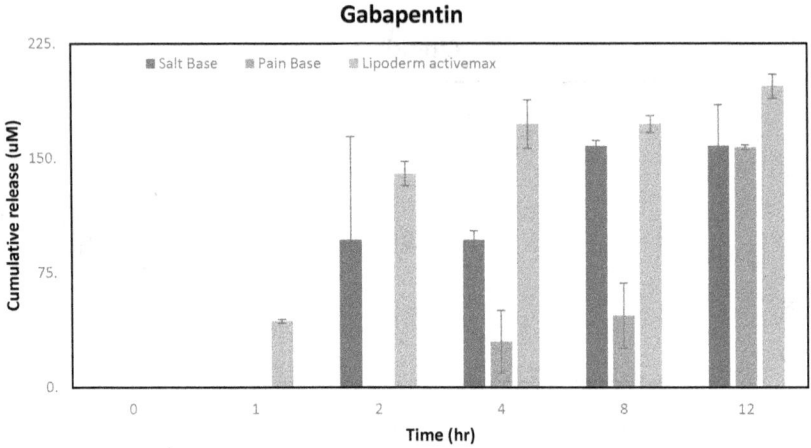

Gabapentin

Cumulative release (uM) vs *Time (hr)*

■ Salt Base ■ Pain Base ■ Lipoderm activemax

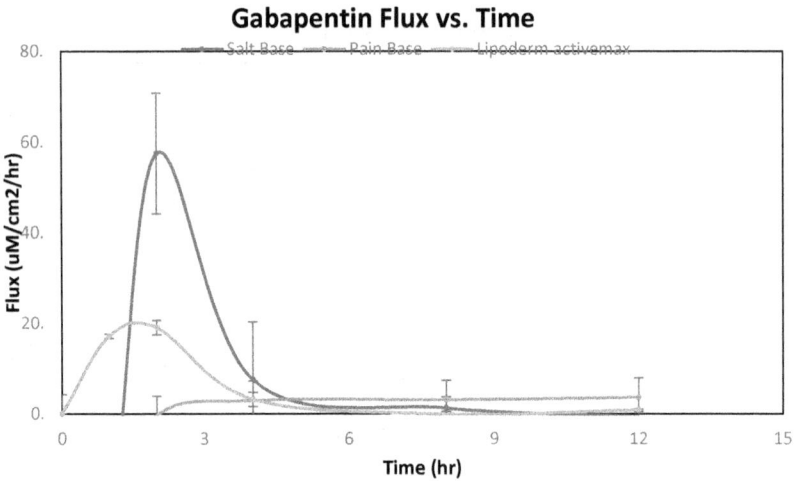

Gabapentin Flux vs. Time

Salt Base —— Pain Base —— Lipoderm activemax

Flux (uM/cm2/hr) vs *Time (hr)*

Lidocaine

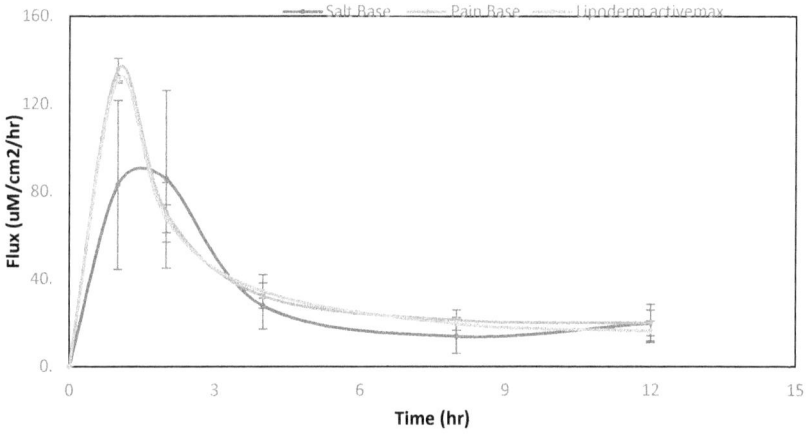

Lidocaine

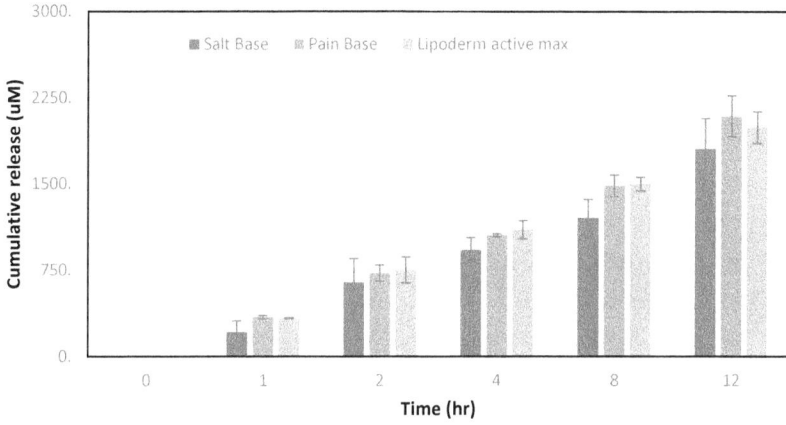

Lidocaine Flux vs. Time

This rare study showed the ability of these transdermal bases to transfer six active ingredients simultaneously into the patient through a topical application. This also introduced me to the exciting field of being a pharmacist and a researcher. There are further plans for us to study this treatment and its effectiveness in various types of pain disorders. Having this information was relatively unique in that previous studies often used only a few ingredients at best. More active ingredients that independently act on the nerve that transmits the pain signal to the brain mean more pain relief. The study also showed that not all bases deliver all active ingredients the same way, but overall, we see delivery of the ingredients through the skin.

Equally important are the wound care ingredients: phenytoin, misoprostol, nifedipine, honey, and aloe vera. Various commercially available bases are used for this purpose, such as Spirawash, Polyox, Pracasil, and Occlusaderm. I have coauthored a brief article with Dr. Ritter on the basic ingredients used in these creams for use as a primer that other medical professionals can reference. (MacKenzie G. et al. The Value of Pharmaceutical Compounding, [www.rehab-magazine,ca] *Rehab and Community Care*, Fall 2013, 14-17)

Keep in mind that compounding for pain is prescription medication. That means that you need to have a doctor on board to write a prescription. This can be a challenge unless your doctor has already had a positive experience with at least one patient and cream. Sometimes they want to see a study or two. As a compounding pharmacist, I make it my part-time job to dig up studies that help prove I am following the evidence and that these compounds really do help improve the quality of life for many people with pain.

A study conducted in 2000 (Gammaitoni A et al. Topical Ketamine Gel: Possible Role in Treating Neuropathic Pain. *Pain Med.* 2000 Mar; 1[1]: 97-100), which included just five patients with neuropathic pain, demonstrated that ketamine gel could be a treatment possibility. In 1999, a study using 100 patients showed that ketoprofen applied topically demonstrated uptake into the joints where the cream was applied. (Rolf C et al. Intra-articular absorption and distribution of ketoprofen after topical plaster application and oral intake in 100 patients undergoing knee arthroscopy. *British Society of Rheumatology.* 1999;38: 564-567) This was key to demonstrating that this active ingredient can make its way from the skin's surface into the space where the pain is originating. In 2005, a study that combined amitriptyline (2%) and ketamine (1%), starting with only 28 subjects, showed pain relief in neuropathic pain and minimal systemic absorption. (Lynch ME et al. Topical Amitriptyline and Ketamine in Neuropathic Pain Syndromes: an Open-lab Study. *J. Pain.* 2005 Oct 6[10]: 644-9). In 2010, we saw acknowledgment that topical creams could be tried in patients when adequate pain relief was not achieved through orally administered painkillers or when side effects from this mode of administration were a problem. (Derry S et al. Cochrane Database Syst Rev. 2015 PMID: 26068955) In my experience, both are common, but the latter is the tipping point where an argument for topical medication is best introduced.

In cases where an entire leg or both legs are affected, and we want to avoid a gross application to a wide area of pain and therefore increased chance of side effects from active ingredients, it is important to follow dermatome maps. A dermatome is a ribbon of tissue that is innervated by a given nerve from the spine. The concept of a dermatome is common to those who have had an attack of shingles – a reappearance of the chicken pox virus after it emerges from hiding in the spinal cord. The virus travels along the strip of tissue that the nerve supplies and can affect any part along that strip.

In non-shingles pain, this theory also applies if we can trace the nerve in that dermatome back to the spine and apply the pain cream to the side of the spine at the point where the nerve starts. It doesn't matter how much fat tissue the person has, the tissue at the spine normally presents a short distance between the skin and the nerve and allows a short distance for topically applied active pharmaceutical ingredients to be transmitted and relatively easy access to a door that can block pain transmission. (Jones M. Chronic Neuropathic Pain: Pharmacological Interventions in The New Millennium. A Theory of Efficacy. *IJPC*. Vol 4 No.1 Jan/Feb 2000)

Another productive way to attack pain is to focus on trigger points. A trigger point is a point of origin of a pain that may actually be in a different area. Myofascial pain is the type of pain that originates from these triggers or knots. This pain actually accounts for many complaints of pain from plantar fasciitis to migraines, repetitive strain, fibromyalgia, and most types of soft tissue injury where neck, back, leg, and shoulder pain exist. The point of all this is that when a pain cream is applied to a trigger point, an entire muscle or muscle group can get relief from pain. Knowledge of this map of trigger points and associated pain distribution is key to diagnosing and treating myofascial pain. My favourite common source for learning about trigger points has been the *Winner's Guide to Pain Relief* (Blatman H et al. Danua Press. 2006).

By understanding the types of receptors that various active ingredients work on, we can create an additive effect by combining as many receptors as possible to relieve pain. Ingredients that seemingly may not have anything to do with pain, such as loperamide, guaifenesin, and pentoxifylline, can have beneficial effects in a topically applied pain medication. (Dunteman, E D. Targeted Peripheral Analgesics in Chronic Pain Syndromes. *Practical Pain Management*. 2011; Volume 5, Issue #5) This is because different active ingredients can all work in separate pathways to ultimately reduce pain topically, even when they may be used for another reason when given orally.

Patients with fibromyalgia are all too familiar with trigger points in their pain experience, and years of treatment have taught us that this is not a normal or well-understood disorder. In fact, just getting the diagnosis can be an ordeal. People struggling with fibromyalgia commonly turn to complementary and alternative therapies because of their struggle to find pain solutions that allow them to carry on with daily life. Quite often, I speak with fibromyalgia patients who use acupuncture, massage therapy, meditation, physiotherapy, and TENS (transcutaneous electrical nerve stimulation) devices. It is not uncommon for me to see a fibromyalgia patient who is plagued by side effects or adverse effects of the NSAID, narcotic, or antidepressant they are put on for this disease, which makes topical preparations attractive to them. Antidepressant use for fibromyalgia has shown some benefits in the short term, but long-term prospective studies fail to show benefit. (Jaeschke R, Adachi J, Guyatt G, Keller J, Wong B: Clinical usefulness of amitriptyline in fibromyalgia: the results of 23 N-of-1 randomized controlled trials. *J Rheumatol* 1991, 18: 447–451; and Abeles M, Solitar BM, Pillinger MH, Abeles AM: Update on fibromyalgia therapy. *Am J Med* 2008, 121: 555–561)

In regard to rheumatic diseases, several studies have had equally promising results in efficacy with topically applied active ingredients. The side-effect profile makes this mode of administration significantly more preferable than oral administration. The maximum concentration of an anti-inflammatory in the blood of the patient following administration of a topical is typically anywhere under 10% and normally less than 5% of the applied dose, depending on the base used. (Heyneman CA et al, Oral vs Topical NSAIDs in Rheumatic Diseases. *Drugs*. 2000 Sep; 60[3]). Many readings are less than 2%. The absorption into the systemic circulation is slow and generally in small amounts when the topical is applied to intact skin. If there are any side effects to be suspected with these ingredients, I would hypothesize that topical anesthetics may not adapt well to heart issues like arrhythmia when concentrations are 3% or more, or to ketamine in higher concentrations, as it may lead to mild mental confusion. Rash is the most common side effect, with 5% incidence. The enzyme systems in the liver that remove many medications from the body are also found in the tissue, which helps to remove the medications quickly from the body.

Where is the evidence on these compounds? As of late, I have been following some interesting studies with gabapentin, one of the commonly used active ingredients in my pain creams, as well as a commonly prescribed oral pain medication for neuropathic pain. In the March/April 2015 issue of the *International Journal of Pharmaceutical Compounding* (Heustess A. Analgesic Efficacy and Transdermal Penetration of Topical Gabapentin Creams: Finding an Optimal Dose and Pretreatment Time. 2015. Volume 19 #2), a peer-reviewed study demonstrated the absorption into the skin and deeper tissues with gabapentin in a Lipoderm base and its effect on pain relief using hamsters as test subjects. This study demonstrated that pain relief and tissue penetration were achieved with this type of cream, but there seemed to be an optimum dose at 5% rather than 1% or 10% gabapentin when they used flinch response as a pain measurement. Duration of action beyond four hours in this study was not shown, and the authors urged further study in this area. Six percent gabapentin is our normal concentration used in these creams.

When ketamine is used for neuropathic pain and amitriptyline is used for post-herpetic neuralgia, we see favourable results. A study presented at the 2007 American Pain Society annual meeting demonstrated the statistically significant improvement in pain reduction between amitriptyline 4% and ketamine 2% cream compared to placebo. Less than 5% of the subjects had detectable levels in the blood when these medications were applied topically. Overall, the studies that show negative results are often those with smaller percentages of active ingredients, which makes sense.

In June of 2011, a randomized study of 208 patients, using baclofen, amitriptyline, and ketamine in an older type of base called PLO (pluronic lecithin organogel), showed benefits over PLO placebo alone in reducing tingling, cramping, and shooting or burning pain associated with chemotherapy-induced peripheral neuropathy (Barton DL et al. A double-blind, placebo-controlled trial of a topical treatment for chemotherapy-induced peripheral neuropathy. *Support Care Cancer.* 2011 June; 19[6] 833-41), with no toxicity reported.

In a 1998 article (Crowley KL et al. Clinical Application of Ketamine Ointment in the Treatments of Sympathetically Maintained Pain. *IJPC* Mar/Apr 98; p. 122), a small study of five patients found no reported side effects in topically applied ketamine on a 24- and 48-hour follow-up. This brings to light a common question with topicals. Does the use of topicals instead of oral medications result in fewer side effects? Do the active chemicals in topicals appear in the blood? As shown in the above study, detectable levels of the drug were not found when we looked for them in the blood. The same is true of topically applied hormones. Personally, I think the only place that scientists should be looking for topically applied compounds is within the tissue, or perhaps the saliva.

Compounding is a prime example of where a treatment option that is not mainstream is driven not only by the results that I and the physicians I work with see on a regular basis, but also by the patients who return to us and ask for the pain creams to be refilled for them.

In my compounding practice, I tend to use a "shotgun approach" of four or five ingredients rather than just one or two. Because of the cost involved with these creams, I prefer using more ingredients that act on multiple receptors rather than just one with a trial-and-error approach. Perhaps someone may get sufficient pain relief with fewer ingredients or a lower strength of each, but compounding a new product each time is cost-prohibitive for many.

Thank you for allowing me to indulge in my passion of compounded topical medicine. This would hardly be a preventive medicine chapter on pain without discussion of a few supplements and the studies that back them up, so we will finish the chapter with that discussion.

SUPPLEMENTS FOR PAIN

Magnesium deficiency (or at least subclinical deficiency) is not uncommon in western societies. Magnesium deficiency is distinct from clinical hypomagnesemia, a severe deficiency situation. The most common presentation of low magnesium is muscle cramps. Magnesium supplementation has been found to improve muscle cramps in controlled and uncontrolled trials.

Lowered **vitamin D**, which is found in some residents in Canada, the US (Gaby page 109), and other nations farther from the equator, has been shown to be associated with pain. The definition of deficiency varies from lab to lab, but a level of 10-15 ng/ml or 25-37.5 nmol/L of 25(OH)D in the serum (the most frequently used indicator of vitamin D status) is considered to be diagnostic of low vitamin D.

A level of 30 ng/ml is considered by many to be a minimum target. Vitamin D deficiency may be the cause of the muscle pain that causes many people to come off statins, although the lowered magnesium, Co-Q10, and potassium could also be at play.

Higher doses of narcotics are noted in patients with low vitamin D status, and fibromyalgia has been hypothesized to be a vitamin D deficiency disease. (http://www.medscape.com/viewarticle/590151) There have been suggestions that anyone with chronic pain should be screened for their vitamin D status. (http://www.medscape.com/viewarticle/538290)

A study published in 2014 (a randomized placebo-controlled trial), showed that when patients with fibromyalgia were brought from less than 80 nmol/L of vitamin D to above that level, the patients reported less pain from this disease. (Wepner F et al. Effects of Vitamin D on Patients with Fibromyalgia Syndrome: A Randomized Placebo Controlled Trial. *Pain*. Feb 2014; Vol 155[2]; 261-268)

In conclusion, pain can be a huge reason for lack of mobility, increase in prescription and OTC drug load, sleep problems, and mood disorders. It is also important to note that any of these issues can lead to deterioration of our relationships and the general quality of our lives. This should make it obvious why I have included this discussion in this book. Although being pain-free may not be a concept we entertain when it comes to long-term pain, coming to an agreement on expectations and goals with a long-term pain patient can have amazing results. In an era where the realization of opioid issues has come to light, treatment by other means is now more important than ever. There has never been dependence found with using opioids transdermally, and side effects are much less than when taken orally. Initiating a discussion between your physician and a compounding pharmacist can make a huge difference in your health.

HEALTHY LOGIC

CHAPTER 12

HEALTHY GROCERY SHOPPING

"Food is an important part
of a balanced diet."

– FRAN LEBOWITZ

In tying together everything I have discussed thus far, it is important to know how to actually choose your food at the grocery store. I work with patients who are often confused about what to eat or are intimidated by health food stores. Most of the patients I see in the pharmacy discover that the key to improving their health and their weight is to prepare most of their meals at home. In order to cook, you have to go to the grocery store, and you need to know what to shop for.

Most of us don't eat enough whole food like fresh fruits and vegetables. We absorb vitamins, minerals, and phytonutrients best in this natural form. By having a salad or two per day, fruit snacks, or raw veggies with a healthy dip, you can easily get more tasty raw whole foods into your diet.

PRODUCE

One simple way that I like to think about nutrition in produce is by colour. It can be very surprising how patterns of nutrition can be determined by something as simple as pigmentation. Let's take a look:

Greens
Greens are some of the most neglected foods in our diet. Examples include spinach, kale, collard greens, mustard greens, Swiss chard, arugula, and romaine lettuce.

Here are some advantages to eating greens and a few tips on their preparation:

- Loaded with nutrients such as calcium, magnesium, zinc, vitamins A, C, E, & K, fibre, and chlorophyll. (Be cautious if on blood thinners as vitamin K-rich greens can counter their effects.)
- Feed the immune system nutrients so it is working at its best. (Note: it doesn't "boost" the immune system.)

- Good for bone health.
- Kale is a nutritional powerhouse, loaded with antioxidants. Only 33 calories per cup. More iron than beef per calorie. Anti-inflammatory with omega-3.
- Toss a handful of spinach or kale in your smoothie.
- Try a spinach salad with walnuts and strawberries or mandarin segments.
- Greens are very easy to cook. Steam in a pan with a little hot water, or sauté with olive oil, onions, and garlic.
- Splash a little vinegar or lemon juice on the greens to make it easier for the body to absorb the calcium.
- How to make crispy kale: Toss the kale with a small amount of olive oil, spread it on a cookie sheet, sprinkle with garlic salt, and bake at 400 F until browned around the edges. Or sauté with a bit of olive oil and garlic.
- Chard sautés easily with a little olive oil. You can add tomato sauce or splash some vinegar onto it and add nuts and raisins.

Red, Orange, and Yellow Produce

Red fruits and vegetables include radishes, red peppers, pomegranates, tomatoes, strawberries, apples, cherries and watermelon, which are all high in nutrients and phytochemicals.

Orange fruits and vegetables include oranges, carrots, orange peppers, yams, and sweet potatoes. Health benefits:

- Help vision, bone growth, healthy skin, and cardiovascular system.
- Contain beta-carotene, vitamin A, vitamin C, potassium, fibre, folate, antioxidants, and phytochemicals.

Bake sweet potatoes with olive oil and cinnamon and eat at the end of your meal. They taste like dessert, with a pumpkin-pie texture.

To make sweet potato fries, cut sweet potatoes into strips and bake at 400 degrees F for 30–35 minutes.

Yellow fruits and vegetables (yellow squash, lemons, yellow peppers).

- Use freshly squeezed lemon juice when making soup stocks. The acid will help leach calcium from chicken and meat bones, making a calcium-rich broth.
- Chop organic peppers, onions, squash, and carrots and roast with olive oil for one hour, turning occasionally, for a delicious vegetable dish that can be reheated for days.
- Keep lemons on hand to add flavour and for cleaning.

White produce (onions, garlic, artichokes, fennel, parsnips, ginger, cauliflower).

Onions, garlic, and ginger are antibacterial, antifungal, and high in phytochemicals.

Purple or Blue produce (eggplant, beets, purple cabbage, blueberries, blackberries).

- Rich in antioxidants, fibre, and vitamin C.
- Prevent early signs of aging and heart disease.
- Beets are high in sugar as well so are great for sugar cravings and are high in iron and folate. Great steamed or sliced, or you can roast them in the oven with olive oil and sea salt or put them in salads.

Root Vegetables

Colours can be a useful tool, but let's look at some other ways to classify produce. Root vegetables are delicious and are full of essential nutrients. They are high in fibre and have a lot of sugar, which makes them great for reducing sugar cravings for treats. Keep in mind, however, that the sugars found in these vegetables, especially carrots, potatoes, beets, and squash, have a higher glycemic index and can make it difficult to lose weight if consumed all together or in excess.

Cruciferous Vegetables

Vegetables from this group, which include cabbage, broccoli, brussels sprouts, radishes, cress, bok choy, and kale, should be eaten on a regular basis. These vegetables have a compound that helps to create a favourable estrogen metabolite balance in women and men. They are also rich in fibre and help to reduce cholesterol levels.

Sea Vegetables

You may not be quite as familiar with this group. Why would anyone want to eat sea vegetables? Sea vegetables offer the broadest range of minerals of any food, containing B vitamins and virtually all the minerals in the ocean – which are the same minerals found in human blood. There are over 75 species commonly eaten around the world.

Sea Vegetables contain vitamins, minerals, and protein, yet are very low in calories. Most of us unknowingly consume sea vegetables as thickeners and stabilizers in foods such as ice cream, instant pudding, salad dressings, and even toothpaste. They are great in stews, soups, salads, or stir-fries. You can eat them as is, but soaking will usually improve their digestibility. Save the soaking water for cooking soups and grains and for watering plants (a great natural fertilizer). Common sea vegetables include nori strips (used for sushi and good for wounds), wakame (used in miso soup), dulse, and kombu.

BEANS, PEAS, AND LENTILS

Beans, peas, and lentils are an excellent source of vegetable protein. They also provide fibre and complex carbohydrates. They're delicious, nutritious, and inexpensive; plus they are easy to cook on the stove or in a slow cooker if you're working all day. And storage is easy – you can keep dried peas, beans, and lentils in an airtight container in your pantry (not in the refrigerator). Soups with beans are easy to make and store well in the fridge or freezer. Adzuki beans are sweeter and easier to digest than other beans, so you may want to consider trying them. Look for adzuki beans in your regular grocery store or bulk food store. Specialty food stores quite often carry them too.

PROTEIN

Now that we have a strong handle on the produce department, let's take a look at other sources of protein, in addition to the beans, peas, and lentils just mentioned.

Nuts and Seeds
In a recent large study in the *New England Journal of Medicine*, researchers at Harvard University looked at how eating nuts may help reduce the risk of mortality, finding that both males and females who ate nuts such as pistachios, almonds, walnuts, hazelnuts, cashews, pecans, and Brazil nuts every day saw health benefits accrue as the consumption of nuts increased. The study authors concluded that "the findings from our study and others suggest a potential benefit of nut consumption for promoting health and longevity."

Pistachios make a great everyday healthy snacking choice for people striving for seven servings a week. Pistachios are a deliciously simple way to snack healthily. A one-ounce serving of pistachios equals approximately 49 nuts, which is more nuts per serving than any other snack nut, and a reduced serving of about 30 pistachios is just about 100 calories. A naturally cholesterol-free food, ninety percent of the fat in pistachios is the healthy unsaturated type. It's easy to spot the good nutrition provided by pistachios, the colorful nut, which owe their green, yellow, and purple-red colors to the antioxidants and polyphenols found in the kernels and skins. Pistachios are a great-tasting, convenient, and healthy snack providing protein, fibre, and antioxidants.

All nuts are seeds, but all seeds are not nuts.

Almonds are a good snack and they're a good source of protein and calcium. Sesame seeds are very rich in calcium as well and are great sprinkled onto salads or greens. They are high in phytosterols, help to lower cholesterol, and contain potassium and magnesium to help lower blood pressure.

The top five seeds and nuts to eat if you are trying to lower cholesterol are: sunflower seeds, pistachios, pumpkin seeds, pine nuts, and whole flaxseeds, freshly ground.

Nuts are not only incredibly delicious and rich tasting, but they are full of good-quality fats that trigger the hormone ghrelin, produced in the stomach to signal your brain that you are full and satisfied.

One of the reasons that fats in nuts are high-quality is that they are anti-inflammatory, which means they fight inflammation, which is key to fighting off many diseases like heart disease and arthritis, Just don't go nuts on the portion size, since fat has the highest calorie density (nine calories per gram of fat). So, for a 100-calorie snack, count out about twelve almonds, ten hazelnuts, four macadamia nuts, or two Brazil nuts.

Keep in mind when you're cooking with nuts or adding them to a recipe that most recipes contain other fat sources, so keep an eye on the portion size of other fatty ingredients such as cheese, oils, and avocado, and scale back accordingly.

Fish

Most people are aware of the benefits of eating fish. Fatty, oily fish are high in omega-3 fatty acids. Examples of omega-3-rich fish include mackerel, lake trout, sardines, albacore tuna, and salmon. However, albacore ("white tuna") has more mercury than canned light tuna. Some recommendations are no more than one serving of albacore tuna per month, based on your age.

The Canadian government recommends that we try to eat at least three servings of fish per week. Salmon, trout, herring, haddock, canned light tuna, pollack, sole, flounder, anchovy, char, hake, mullet, smelt, mackerel, and lake white fish have the lowest levels of contaminants. Higher levels of methyl mercury are found in fresh and frozen tuna, shark, swordfish, and marlin. This is especially important in pregnancy. Be sure to check local advisories on recommendations in your area.

Omega-3 is important for reducing inflammation. This benefits everyone and especially those with heart disease, eye disease, high cholesterol, and even arthritis. It also protects against blood clots, lowers triglycerides, raises HDL, and prevents heart arrhythmias.

It's important to buy good-quality fish. In a regular grocery store, you'll want to read labels and talk to the counter person. Look for wild, fresh-caught fish. Wild fish grow in natural environments and eat plankton and krill, which converts to omega-3. Their diverse diets give them their natural coloring and higher nutritional value. In contrast, be cautious with farmed fish. Farmed fish are fed pellets. They are also often fed colourings to make them look more enticing when brought to market. Farmed fish are raised very closely together in pens, creating a higher chance of disease. They may be fed antibiotics to counter disease or hormones to make them grow faster and bigger. A good trick for finding "fresh" fish is to ask if you can smell it. If it smells fishy, it's probably not that fresh.

Smaller, non-predatory fish that swim closer to the surface contain less mercury. Try to stick to fish that can fit in a large frying pan. Canned fish is a great item to keep in the pantry for a quick dinner. Salmon, sardines (a great source of calcium), and anchovies are all great in pastas and salads.

For scallops, farmed is the best way to go. Wild scallops are traditionally harvested by dredging, which causes environmental damage. Buy scallops labeled "dry"; otherwise, they've been treated with sodium tripolyphosphate. This is put on the scallop to absorb up to 50 percent of its weight in water and is claimed to be a preservative by the industry. Canada has limits on the total level allowed in seafood products, but some countries don't have limits at all. This is the biggest case of consumer fraud in the seafood industry.

Meat

A lot of people enjoy eating meat. Ideally, look for antibiotic-free and hormone-free meat. Most of us eat too much meat. In meat, "organic" means that the animal was given only 100% organic feed without ground-up animal parts. It also means the animal was not given antibiotics, growth hormones, or other drugs. Free range or graze means the animals were raised in humane conditions. They were allowed to spend time outdoors in the fresh air and had access to a natural food source such as grass for cows and bugs for chickens, the most ideal food for them.

CARBOHYDRATES

In recent years, diet fads have swung toward the concept of low-carb diets. Sugars have come to be recognized as one of the primary drivers of obesity, and books like *Wheat Belly* have caused a cultural sensation that has made much of our population wary of eating bread and pasta. Of course, the key with carbohydrates, as with all things, is moderation.

NATURAL SWEETENERS

A great alternative to refined, processed, empty-calorie sweeteners are natural sweeteners. Unrefined sweeteners generally contain more flavour, and they undergo minimal processing techniques. Keep in mind, though, that sugar is sugar. They are very concentrated, so a little goes a long way, and they still should only be used in moderation. Raw honey and maple syrup quickly enter the bloodstream, so they are great for a quick energy boost. Sweeteners such as barley malt and brown rice syrup enter the bloodstream at a much slower rate, which is a great alternative for those who want or need to avoid sugar. Each one has their own flavour and sweetness level.

Some samples of natural sweeteners are:

- Honey – can be helpful for allergy symptoms; will affect blood sugar levels; raw honey has natural enzymes; don't give to children under the age of two
- Maple syrup – contains minerals and enzymes; also affects blood sugar levels
- Barley malt – tastes similar to molasses; use for baking or to sweeten tea; enters the blood stream slowly
- Brown rice syrup – smooth, buttery flavour; enters the blood stream slowly
- Stevia – from an herb
- Xylitol – a sugar alcohol; inhibits bacteria that causes tooth decay; may cause stomach upset; use in moderation

SUGAR

Sugar is a major cause of inflammation. It can cause hyperglycemia, diabetes, high cholesterol, mood swings, depression, tooth decay, energy crashes, and hormone fluctuation, and contributes to chronic disease. Most processed foods are loaded with sugar, and it's usually the cheapest form – high-fructose corn syrup. Corn syrup is processed by the liver, and excess sugar makes the liver fatty.

As a rule of thumb, there are four grams of sugar per teaspoon, which is equal to one packet of sugar. One 12-oz can of soda has approximately 40 grams of sugar. That is almost ten teaspoons of sugar in one can of soda.

Fruit juice, fruit drinks, and vitamin water are not any better, which is why I removed all of these beverages from my pharmacy in 2014. It was a move that generated a lot of attention nationally and beyond. My pharmacy sales increased both in the pharmacy and front shop afterward, which I have always attributed to this move. As a result of this removal, a Canadian scientist by the name of Dr. Leia Minaker picked up on the story and decided to conduct a "natural study" to determine the effects of one store not selling these sugary beverages in a small town where there were only a few sources of sugary beverages. Leia works at the Propel Centre for Population Health Impact at the University of Waterloo in Ontario, Canada. At this centre, they lead and stimulate relevant and rigorous studies that can move evidence into action to make a healthier country. The study was published in *BMC Public Health* (Minaker et al. *BMC Public Health*. 2016; 16:586).

Dr. Minaker and her group analyzed our data of total product sales from January 1, 2013, to May 8, 2015. The grocery and convenience stores in my town were good enough to supply their data of carbonated sugared beverages for the same period. The graph below shows the results:

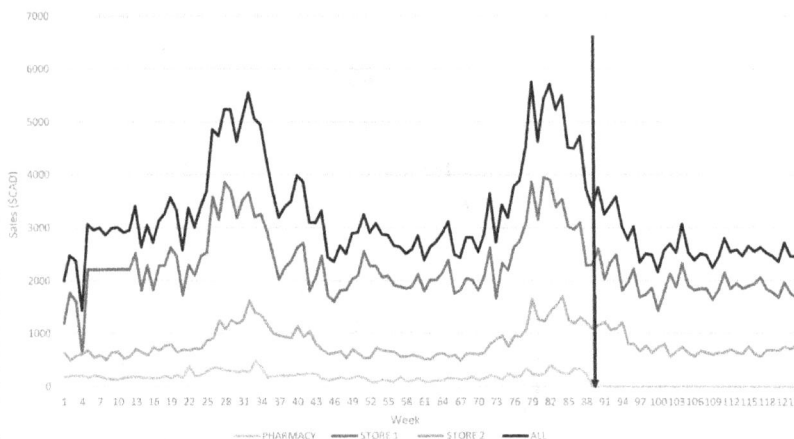

Fig. 1 Weekly sales ($CAD) of carbonated soft drinks, Baddeck, Nova Scotia, January 1, 2013 to May 8, 2015. The black arrow represents time of policy introduction. Carbonated soft drinks include diet and regular varieties

At week 89, we stopped selling the sugary beverages (carbonated sugary beverages, all juice, sports drinks, chocolate milk, and vitamin water). It was a shock to many who thought that drinking juice was healthy, which it is not.

As Dr. Minaker explains, this study was among the first to examine the impact of a restrictive food environment policy on carbonated soft drink (CSD) sales at the community level. Several limitations should be noted. First, there was no control community, and there has been a gradual decline over the past few years in CSD sales in the province of Nova Scotia. However, the decline in CSD sales at a provincial level was not as dramatic as the declines observed in the current study. Second, it is possible that people living in my small town of Baddeck would drive out of town to buy their soft drinks. However, given that the nearest larger centre is about forty minutes' drive away, and given that these drinks were still available in both the grocery store and the convenience stores, it is unlikely that there was an increase in out-of-town CSD procurement. In fact, the lack of switching behaviour in buying more sugary drinks from another local store suggests that the community may indeed have gotten the message on the campaign. Finally, the most significant limitation of the current study was the relatively short follow-up time (35 weeks post-policy). It is likely that the lack of statistical significance accompanying the estimates was caused by the short follow-up time. Another reason for the lack of statistical significance was likely the large standard errors caused by the weekly variation in CSD sales.

These limitations, however, are to be expected in a real-world setting and are offset by the fact that all three food stores in the town agreed to share their weekly CSD sales data over a 123-week period. We hope that the current study provides fodder for conversations about the implications of selling health-damaging food products (e.g., sugar-sweetened beverages) in healthcare settings such as pharmacies. As a novel area for population health intervention research, this area of inquiry would benefit from future multi-disciplinary, action-oriented research. For example, legal scholars could examine whether the legal reasoning used to create provincial legislation to prohibit tobacco pharmacy sales could be analogous to legal arguments for prohibiting SSB sales in pharmacies. Business experts could examine and estimate the financial impact of voluntary CSD sales bans in pharmacies and could begin to explore the reputational and social risks of CSD sales for different pharmacy chain brands. Finally, it would be interesting to examine the impact of this type of restrictive food retail intervention on the actual dietary intake of residents, which would require population health researchers to collaborate with practicing community pharmacists to undertake an evaluation of such a policy.

Finally, in comparing the local sales data with the pooled sales data in pop sales in the province of Nova Scotia, a very interesting result was found. The mean increase in pop sales from the two time frames of June 2013 to June 2014 and from June 2014 to June 2015 was 19.4% in a sampling of sales data from 35 pharmacies in the province.

It wasn't until the story of Dr. Minaker's natural study hit the papers five months after the original withdrawal that a second wave of press came out. As a result of that exposure, an editorial in my local paper was published by a senior position holder of a company with an interest in the sugary beverage industry. It basically claimed that my move to not sell these beverages sent the wrong message, that these beverages were wrongly to blame for increasing weight. While I fought the urge to fire back with my own editorial, my thoughts were clear.

In response to my decision to remove sugary drinks from my pharmacy in September of 2014, there seems to be the odd lingering claim out there that targeting the sale of one particular category is not going to have a significant impact on obesity, and that information – not restriction – is key.

While we agree with the point that obesity is a complex, multifactorial problem, it is completely baseless – in fact hovering on outright deception – to claim that extra calorie intake does not increase weight. In 2013, the journal *PLOS Medicine* published a systematic review of systematic reviews, which are the most comprehensive forms of evidence that we have. This review by Bes-Rastrollo and colleagues entitled "Financial Conflicts of Interest and Reporting Bias Regarding the Association between Sugar-Sweetened Beverages and Weight Gain: A Systematic Review of Systematic Reviews," found that 83% of reviews not funded by the beverage industry demonstrated a relationship between sugar-sweetened beverage consumption and weight gain. On the other hand, 83% of the reviews that were funded by the industry found insufficient evidence to support a positive association between sugar-sweetened beverage consumption and weight gain or obesity.

Metabolic disease has also been shown to increase with consumption of these drinks. Metabolic disease is one of the main reasons that pharmacists see customers for high blood pressure, increased cholesterol, increased abdominal obesity, and insulin resistance.

A 2010 meta-analysis in the *Journal of Diabetes Care* that followed over 300,000 subjects found that those who consumed the most sugary drinks, averaging one or two per day (pop, juice, vitamin water, iced tea, or energy drinks), had a 26% greater chance of developing type 2 diabetes than those who drank no sugary drinks or only about one per month. They concluded that weight gain and metabolic syndrome correlate positively with consumption of these drinks. *The New England Journal of Medicine* published a study in 2011 that followed over 120,000 people and concluded that people who consumed one 12-ounce sugary beverage serving a day weighed more than those who did not consume this beverage. Finally, a 2012 study in *Circulation* followed 40,000 men and found a 20% higher chance of having a heart attack or dying from a heart attack when one can of sugary beverage per day was consumed, compared to men who didn't consume any. This was verified by a second study.

Calorie consumption from all sugary beverages combined has continued to climb each decade, especially among children and teens. The World Health Organization has changed its recommendation for daily consumption of sugar to a maximum of 6 to 10 teaspoons daily. This would be exceeded by consuming even one can of soda. Finally, we are seeing revised guidelines on sugar that follow science. The new recommendation advises restricting free sugars to as low as 5% of total calories, meaning a serving of orange juice is off limits. Free sugars are the sugar no longer inside the cells of the fruit, in other words, in fruit juice. Imagine a recommendation that pushes you to eat the fruit instead of drinking the juice. Brilliant! There is now a separation of total sugars and free sugars. The total sugar concept meant you could gobble up your calories with juice and pop, but now it's considered free sugar instead, with a strict recommendation on maximum consumption.

The withdrawal of sugary beverages from Stone's Pharmasave in Baddeck was not meant to "ban" pop sales, and I certainly do not expect to see a drastic change in obesity levels in my town as a result of my decision. I made this decision to help educate my customers on the effects of sugary drinks. I agree that education is an important component of healthy eating. However, in keeping with recommendations from world experts in obesity research (2015 *Lancet* Obesity Series), I am also aiming to move beyond education by starting to create an environment in my store that is supportive of healthy food choices. As a pharmacist, I know I shouldn't sell tobacco, no matter what the industry claims. I feel I shouldn't sell sugary beverages, either.

The American Academy of Pediatrics has updated its guidelines to address the rising tide of childhood obesity. It stresses the control of sugary foods that are brought into the home. This control recommends fewer sweetened beverages, especially for young people. It recommends making healthy choices freely visible at home and that parents should act as role models for their dependents.

FLOUR SUBSTITUTES / WHOLE GRAINS / PASTA / BREADS

For a healthier choice, I recommend you go with a whole-grain flour in place of white flour. In making refined white flour, the grains are milled to remove up to 80% of the grain's nutrients, and much of the flavour is lost in the process. Whole-grain flours have more vitamins, minerals, fibre, and flavours. Some people feel organically grown flour has the best flavour. Whole-grain flour must be refrigerated in moisture-free, tight containers and used within two to four months of purchase. There are many different choices you can experiment with. Favourites include whole-wheat flour, quinoa flour, brown rice flour, oat flour, kamut, spelt, amaranth, barley, millet, potato, teff, and corn.

I recommend you look for sprouted grain and sprouted grain flours. Grains are seeds. Sprouting means the grain has been changed from a seed into a living plant. This happens by allowing the grain to soak in brine long enough to wake it from dormancy. This sets the process of germination into motion. When a grain changes from a seed into a living plant, its nutritional qualities improve, as well as our body's ability to digest it and absorb nutrients. The stored-up nutrients held in the seed burst forth and give life to the sprout. This sprouted grain contains many active enzymes that aid in digestion. Extra vitamin C is produced through sprouting. Vitamin levels such as B1, B2, B3, B5, B6, E, K, and beta-carotene are higher. Phytic acid is also neutralized in sprouted grains, which allows for easier absorption of calcium, magnesium, iron, copper, and zinc. Grains contain lignans, which contain powerful agents that may assist in cancer and heart disease prevention and help maintain bone strength.

It's better to choose good carbs than no carbs, and whole grains are your best bet. They provide energy and are important for a healthy diet. Refined grains on their own or in flour, pasta, or bread are digested too quickly and impact our blood sugar levels. Also, when buying bread, avoid hydrogenated or partially hydrogenated oils and high-fructose corn syrup.

Unfortunately, multigrain products often have bleached flour blended with them in manufacturing. If multigrain isn't the first ingredient, then white flour is most likely the main ingredient. If a company produces real multigrain bread, it will list the actual grains that make up the blend. If not, the blend could contain mostly white flour. Also be cautious of white starch, such as potato starch, listed after the multigrain.

CEREAL

Keeping in line with grains, there are some healthy alternatives to foods that you probably already eat. Breakfast really is the most important meal of the day. Studies show that people who eat breakfast have better concentration, are more easily able to control their weight, and perform better in athletic competitions. A lot of adults and children like to eat cereal. You want to look for a cereal that's made with whole grains and is high in fibre. The recommended intake of fibre per day is about 25 grams (21–38 g). The average Canadian consumes about 14 grams of fibre. Women who consume more fibre are half as likely to be obese.

Look for a cereal that has at least five grams of fibre per serving. One thing to be careful of is the sugar content – ideally a cereal should have five grams of sugar or less. You may notice that after you eat a very sugary, processed cereal, you get hungry again rather quickly, or your energy levels seem like they're great but then dramatically plummet. You can limit these side effects by decreasing the amount of sugar in your cereal.

Watch portion sizes. Many people can easily eat two or three servings of cereal at a sitting before getting full, which is often more than they had planned on eating. Consider premeasuring your cereal so that you don't overeat, especially if that cereal has a high sugar content. A key point in healthy eating is to eat slowly and chew food fully. This can be especially tough at breakfast when everyone is in a hurry.

Also, watch out for high-fructose corn syrup, which is an unhealthy component to many packaged cereals, especially high-fibre cereals. It is added to the fibre cereals because people don't like the taste of fibre. It is also listed as HFCS or "corn sugar."

FIBRE

Fibre comes in two forms: soluble and insoluble. Soluble fibre lowers cholesterol and regulates blood sugar levels. Soluble fibre is found in foods such as oatmeal, oat bran, beans, dried peas, lentils, and pectin-rich foods like apples, strawberries, and citrus fruits. Insoluble fibre, such as that found in wheat bran, whole-grain foods, and the skins, leaves, and seeds of fruits and vegetables, is a bulky roughage that helps you feel full and promotes regularity. As a shortcut, look for 100% whole grain or 100% whole wheat, with wheat germ listed as the first ingredient.

There are lots of ways to increase the fibre in your diet. Just add one more vegetable or one more piece of fruit per day; add beans or lentils to salad, spaghetti sauce, or soup; choose bread or pasta that has high fibre; add a quarter cup of wheat bran, oat bran, or flax to baking; or use hummus or other bean dips for spreads on sandwiches instead of mayo.

DAIRY

It's no secret that some people are allergic or sensitive to cow's milk in some way, either through lactose intolerance or sensitivity to the protein in dairy milk, but aren't sure what to put on their cereal. Canada's food guide has recently changed. One of the issues I had with the old Canada's Food Guide is that there were mandatory servings of dairy per day. The plain truth is that you really do not need to consume milk to be a healthy growing child – or an adult either, for that matter. There is now a revised guide that straightens this out after listening to healthcare professionals in the country. Not that milk is dangerous, just that it's not as necessary as we were led to believe growing up.

Milk alternatives don't contain cow's milk, and usually, they don't carry the same amount of protein or calcium as milk either. There are nut milks, rice milks, oat milks, grain milks, and soy milks. These are made by mixing nuts, grains, or soybeans with water. They mix the water and food choice together, then they strain out the rice, nuts, or whatever, and what you have left over is the milk. Look for unsweetened versions, although the rice milks have natural sugars from the rice, so they are naturally sweeter.

Nut-based milk products are a great milk alternative. They are great in cereals, smoothies, and any recipe that calls for milk.

Goat milk and its products like goat cheese are easier on the digestive system than cow's milk.

Keep in mind that mass-produced yogurt often has little value. High sugar content makes most popular yogurt products less healthy than they should be.

CANADA'S FOOD GUIDE

The Canada Food Guide had its origins around war time in the 1940s and reflected country's overall needs at the time. It tried to strike a balance between what was needed for the war while also addressing the poor health of potential recruits at the time. As the Guide evolved over the decades, the Dairy Bureau of Canada, the Canadian Meat Council, and the Canadian Egg Marketing Agency have all had their input into the guide in a way that increased recommendations for their products. This is not the best way to improve the health of a nation.

One of Canada's most outspoken obesity experts, Dr. Yoni Freedhoff, said in a CBC story back in 2006 that following the old guide could cause weight gain. He is especially critical in the way servings of fruits and vegetables are handled, as well as potential dangers of trans fat, salt, and overeating. Fruit and vegetable servings could be all fruit if you took it literally and should not include fruit juice (even "100%" juice, because that means nothing), and a recommendation to limit your trans fat should read "no trans fat at all."

EGGS

Eggs are a great source of vitamin D. There is no difference in nutritional value between brown eggs and white eggs; they are just laid by different types of hens. Eggs are healthy to eat in moderation. Look for free range, vegetarian fed, and local. Omega-3 eggs are highly perishable and can spoil quicker. Keep in mind that there is a difference between organic and free-range eggs. Organic follows stricter guidelines than conventional free range does, with the primary difference being the chickens are fed an organic diet. Under both titles, the amount of time outdoors is variable, but the animals at least have access to outdoors and are cage-free.

Salmonella contamination has been shown to be lower in cage-free hens in both conventional and organic settings. Pasture-raised or free-range hens generally spend more time outside and eat in grassy areas with insects as food in addition to their feed. They aren't necessarily organic, though. There is generally less crowding in these situations and less disease and healthier immune systems. The birds can engage in more natural behaviours like dust bathing to clean themselves.

In summary, all-natural, cage-free, free-range, pasture-raised, and organic all mean different things. The most nutritious eggs come from birds raised outside of cages, fed outdoors, and especially from those that have been fed organically, as this leads to the highest levels of omega-3 in the eggs.

A 2013 review of 16 separate studies on the issue of eggs and cardiovascular disease found that there was no increased risk of heart disease in healthy people eating an egg a day compared to those who rarely or never ate eggs. However, the review also found that high egg consumption was associated with an increased risk of coronary heart disease in type 2 diabetics. Of course, type 2 diabetics are already at increased risk of heart disease.

This shows that the case for eggs is not as black and white as some may believe and may have as much to do with the person eating the egg as the egg itself. Overall, a moderate intake of free-range eggs is likely fine for most healthy people.

CONDIMENTS & SPICES

Condiments and spices are an excellent opportunity to add flavour and variety in a healthy way when preparing meals. These can be used with casseroles, vegetables, soups, whole grains, salads, and more. Many are healthy and low calorie.

Salty – Tamari, Mustard. These give a lot of flavour without adding fat or calories and aid in digestion. They are antifungal, antibacterial, antiseptic, and anti-inflammatory.

Sour – Apple Cider Vinegar, Balsamic Vinegar, Lemons, and Limes. Apple cider vinegar is great on greens and in lentil and bean soups. It's antibacterial and antifungal. I often recommend increasing acid for those with reflux disease, as it helps aid in digestion and enzyme activation. Increased acid also helps with absorption of minerals such as calcium in greens. Balsamic vinegar is a sweeter form of vinegar that is great on roasted vegetables and salads. Lemons and limes are delicious on vegetables, fish, poultry, greens, and soups.

Spicy – Chilies, Cayenne pepper, Red Pepper Flakes, Hot Sesame Seed Oil, Mustard, Ketchup, and Barbeque Sauce. Chilies are a personal favourite of mine because they provide a spark of flavour and a flash of heat to foods that would otherwise be bland. Eating spicy, flavourful food can also help you feel full without eating large portions. They also have the added bonus of a reduced calorie and fat intake in the short term. Chilies are a champion spice because they are extremely low in calories; are fat-free, salt-free and sugar-free; and are a good source of vitamins A, C, and E, folate, and potassium. Capsaicin, which gives hot peppers their hotness, has been studied for its ability to stimulate circulation and ease the pain of arthritis. The best way to incorporate chilies into your diet is to buy them fresh and use them in healthy, home-cooked meals.

Nutty – Nut Butters. There are lots of different varieties of nut butters. Almond butter is a great choice. Tahini, a popular product made from ground sesame seeds, is full of calcium and great when making hummus or on salads or vegetables.

Cloves – Great as a spice, linked to anti-inflammatory properties and pain relief.

TEA & COFFEE

Tea is the most consumed beverage in the world after water. **Black, green, and red teas** are all high in antioxidants, and studies have linked these teas to a lower risk of cancer, blood clots, and high cholesterol levels. Green and black tea have ten times the antioxidants of fruits and vegetables, promote digestion, and contain high amounts of polyphenols. They protect cells from free radicals. Drink at least two cups daily to maximize health benefits.

Herbal teas are not made from tea leaves. They are made with herbs, flowers, roots, spices, grasses, nuts, barks, and botanicals. Herbal teas are great for relaxation, digestion, sleep, colds, and other ailments. You can drink them hot or iced, and there's a large selection available to experiment with.

Coffee. For people who are trying to eliminate or reduce their caffeine intake, there are many great coffee alternatives available, such as herbal coffees, or those made from grains, nuts, chicory, fruit, or mushrooms.

As always, if you are willing to spend some extra money, look for Fair Trade certifications, which indicate that the coffee farmers and workers have been treated fairly.

There are no shortage of Media stories out there quoting studies of the month that claim coffee is good or bad for you. These claims involve benefits with respect to cancer, parkinsonism, liver and heart health and more. Also, decaf coffee appears to have no adverse health effects. My favourite stance on coffee is since new claims are hard to keep track of, we would probably know at this point if it were killing us. Drink away!

SNACK FOODS

This is where most healthy eating falls apart. Everyone likes chips, crackers, or other snack food occasionally. These types of foods should be eaten only occasionally and in moderation, if at all. Look for snacks that are free of artificial colors and flavours, artificial sweeteners, and hydrogenated oils and trans fats. Be careful of products that appear to be "health food store oriented." Vitamin water, for example, is not much different from a soft drink. It is mainly sugary water. Often, we find HFCS or aspartame in these drinks. Most vitamin drinks are not actually healthy at all.

Aspartame itself has not been found to have a harmful effect on health at levels most humans would consume, despite the fact that many try to avoid using it as a sweetener due to claims it causes cancer, diabetes, or other health issues. It has been found, however, that it isn't as effective in promoting weight loss as reported in 2017 by the Canadian Medical Association. Another example is "healthy" potato chips, many of which are still fried, although probably in a healthier oil. Studies are also linking all fried foods to long-term health risks, and foods like this are still high in fat and calories, so they do not support our bodies being healthy. Some baked chips are available instead of fried. Compare labels. You will likely find significantly less fat in baked chips, but much more sugar and the same amount of salt as in fried chips. Overall, most chips are low in nutrient value.

FROZEN FOODS

Frozen veggies are great to have on hand for a quick dinner side dish, and frozen fruit is great for dessert or smoothies. Frozen meat and fish are fine, but stick to the guidelines I mentioned earlier (antibiotic-free, hormone-free, wild-caught). There are lots of delicious gluten-free alternatives in the frozen section as well. These are all good for stocking up as convenience and emergency items. It is important to avoid brands that are packaged in plastic trays or need microwaving. The Canadian Cancer Society strongly recommends to never microwave food in plastic due to chemicals that may leach out of the container into the food, which can increase your risk of cancer.

FATS & OILS

Fat is necessary for many reasons, from brain function to vitamin absorption. Healthy fats are essential to good health. Extra virgin oils are the least processed, and we should aim to avoid processed oils. Further, make sure you purchase oils that are stored in a dark glass bottle, as light speeds up rancidity. Also store oils away from heat and light. Be careful not to over-buy oil. Buy what you can use in three months to prevent oxidation.

> **Olive oil** is a healthy source of fat that may reduce the risk of heart disease and other diseases. Buy extra virgin, cold-pressed olive oil. Olive oil is most nutritious when cooked at low temperature to medium heat (375°F). Once an oil smokes or burns, its flavour and nutrient content decrease.

Coconut oil has a high smoke point, which makes it great for cooking. It also requires extra energy to digest, which increases metabolism. Look for virgin or extra virgin and organic. Coconut oil is also great as a skin lotion and is antifungal.

Avocado oil has a very high smoke point – 500 degrees F – and has the highest level of heart-healthy monounsaturated fat of any cooking oil. New studies show it may aid diabetics by improving blood lipids. It also has high levels of omega-9.

Grapeseed oil is good for high-heat cooking, and **sesame oil** is good for low-heat cooking.

CONCLUSION

Hopefully this gives you some ideas about some new foods to try or products to consider. A lot of people get into grocery shopping ruts and buy the same things week after week – or worse, they don't grocery shop at all. Keep in mind that healthy living involves some form of exercise as well as eating right.

Some Final Words of Wisdom

- Do not shop when you're hungry.
- Avoid saturated fat, trans fat, sodium, high-fructose corn syrup, enriched flour, and added sugars.
- Daily protein intake in grams should be 0.8 times your weight in kg.
- Get used to reading nutrition information on packaging. Pay special attention to what a serving size is for that product.

- Centre your meals around fresh vegetables, which should fill at least half of your plate. Include salads with dressings that aren't loaded with calories or unhealthy fat.
- Studies show people eat what's on their plate, so start with smaller plates and serve your salad on a separate salad plate.

Warm thanks to Cheryl Heppard, who helped to assemble parts of our grocery store tour.

www.ingramcontent.com/pod-product-compliance
Lightning Source LLC
Chambersburg PA
CBHW070809270326
41927CB00010B/2367